W E L L N E S S
FOR~EVERY~ONE

*How to create optimal health, happiness
and longevity for the 21st century*

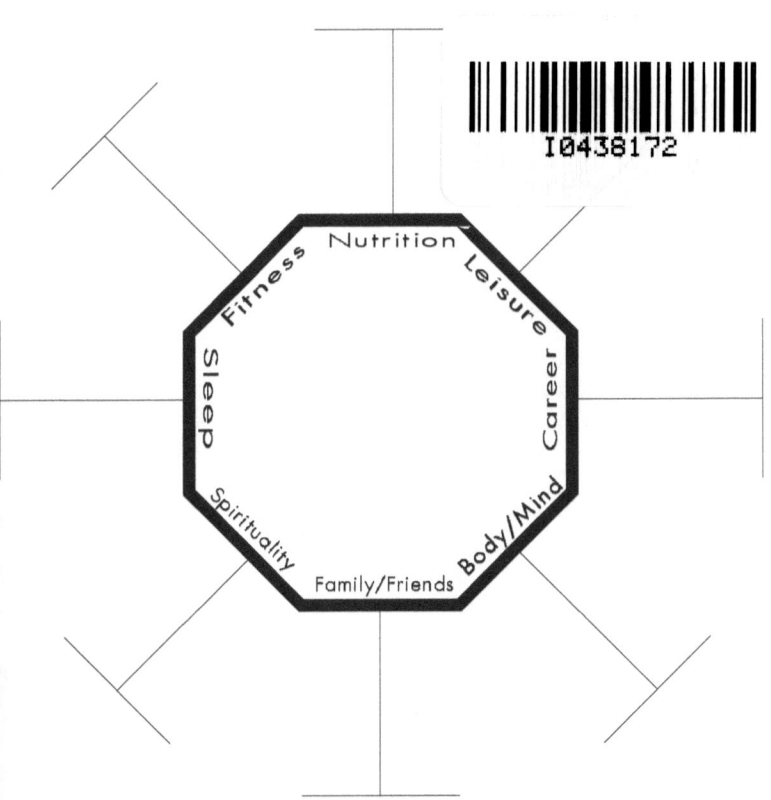

Nutrition

Fitness

Leisure

Sleep

Career

Spirituality

Body/Mind

Family/Friends

WELLNESS
FOR~EVERY~ONE

*How to create optimal health, happiness
and longevity for the 21st century*

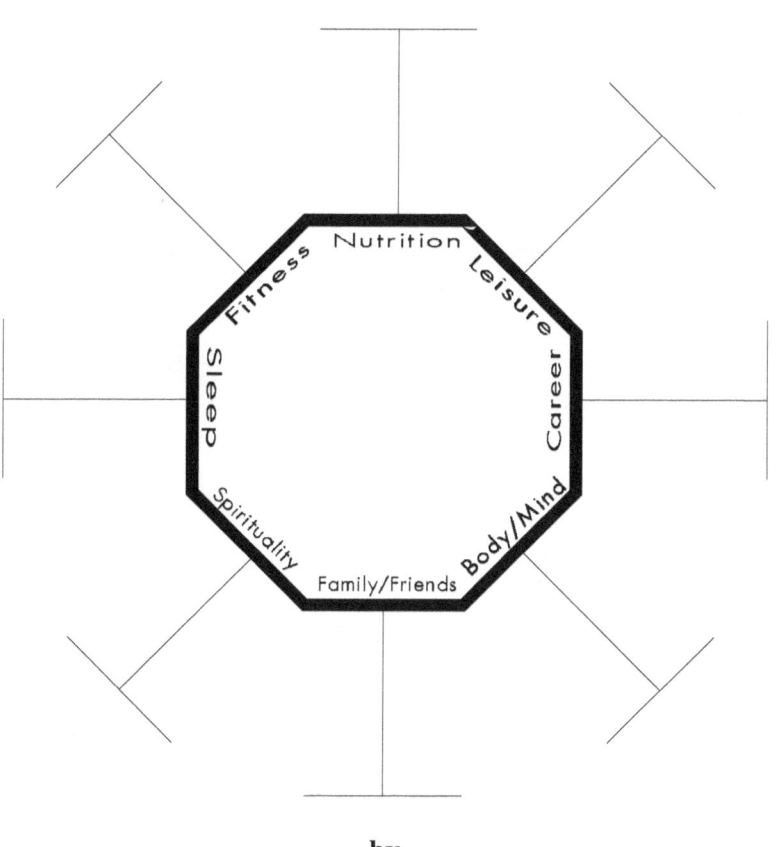

by

JAMES A. DENNIS JR.

Occupational Therapist

ISBN: 978-1-5850-0573-4 (sc)
ISBN: 000-0-0000-0277-4 (e)

Print information available on the last page.

This book is printed on acid-free paper.

1stBooks - rev. 1/8/26

About the Book

Wellness For~Every~One: How to create optimal health, happiness, and longevity for the 21st century, is a concept of synergy. The synergy of wellness can also be described as your whole life. As other books concentrate on specific areas of wellness, this book reveals the eight wellness areas that need to be addressed when learning about this subject. The author has presented a simple and balanced approach by creating a working model which allows the reader to see wellness, to remember what it is, and to understand how each wellness area supports the other parts.

From the beginning, the author places the responsibility of achieving a high level of wellness on the reader. However, his words do not make the reader feel as if wellness is a chore. He empowers the reader by repeatedly suggesting the main point is to expand your wellness wheel, to help it grow larger and larger, and not smaller and smaller. He also provides four "tools" we can use throughout life when making wellness choices. The primary tool he presents throughout the book is to use your intuition--your inner awareness.

Mr. Dennis describes the eight major wellness areas, which he emphasizes there is no one area that is more important than another, as they all equally play a synergistic role in wellness. The eight areas are: Body/Mind, Career, Family/Friends, Fitness, Leisure, Nutrition, Sleep, and Spirituality. There are individual chapters on all of these areas which provide safe, sound, and powerfully effective suggestions to expand each area. These eight areas are followed by chapters on how to make lasting wellness changes, finding the time for wellness, and discovering a way to have wellness forever.

The author has achieved his intention of creating a model that can be applied equally to everyone--forever, as wellness is never-ending. One of the underlying themes is that we are all perfect exactly how we are right now, and yet we can choose to expand our wellness circle to experience greater health, happiness, and longevity.

Inside you will discover how to:
~ Achieve regular sound sleep without drugs
~ Eat and drink your way to wellness
~ Live in a state of happiness
~ Have fun without guilt
~ Find your bliss career
~ Give love freely to your family and friends
~ Be fit without pain
~ Let your body and mind work together for optimal health

Wellness For~Every~One is a fun book to read, as the author interjects humorous comments throughout. It is fast reading which is not bogged down with tons of examples or medical terms. James Dennis is an Occupational Therapist, and pulls from his personal experiences while making reference to many authors throughout the book, in order to learn more about specific wellness topics.

Whether you are new to wellness, or even if you are an experienced veteran, you will come away with a smile and a feeling of confidence after reading this book.

This book is dedicated to Doriann and Noelani

"I love you forever"

Acknowledgments

I would like to first acknowledge all of the people I forgot to mention here, as this project was such a synergistic effort, it would be impossible to name everyone. Thank you Dori and Noe for letting me experience the "flow" state while writing this book at various hours of the day and night. A smiling thank you to all of my family and friends for letting me experiment wellness ideas on you.(Even when you didn't know it.) To every professor and teacher that put up with my peculiar learning style of "acting out in class," a loving thank you. Of course I must thank 1stBooks and The Ingram Book Company for trusting in me and my message, and helping to share it with the world. Finally, a special thank you to all of the authors I mention in this book, who all sparked my intuition to follow my bliss.

Disclaimer

No book can serve as a substitute for medical advice, so please consult your doctor for help with specific issues.

CONTENTS

CHAPTER ONE:
Wellness   1
CHAPTER TWO:
Nutrition   15
CHAPTER THREE:
Sleep   25
CHAPTER FOUR:
Spirituality   35
CHAPTER FIVE:
Leisure   49
CHAPTER SIX:
Fitness   55
CHAPTER SEVEN:
Family & Friends   61
CHAPTER EIGHT:
Career   69
CHAPTER NINE:
Body/Mind   77
CHAPTER TEN:
Change   97
CHAPTER ELEVEN:
Time   113
CHAPTER TWELVE:
Longevity   119
Follow Up   135
Appendix   137
Recommended Reading List   141

Introduction

Welcome. For whatever reason you have come to be in possession of this information here today, maybe a friend let you borrow it , or you spontaneously bought it, or you found it rummaging through the rubbish. Whatever the reason, fate, luck, cosmic intervention, it is perfect and on purpose.

Wellness is not merely taking a certain vitamin or a performing a special exercise program. Wellness is you-it is your whole life, and your whole life is synergy. And synergy means that the whole is greater than the sum total of your parts. And how can a book claim to show the way to wellness without delving into all of your parts, not just a few of the parts.

I venture to guess that most authors have created books and programs with the intention of helping as many people as possible, whatever the topic is. I too have this same intention, with one exception, I am confident that this presentation is so simple and balanced that it *can* work for~every~one. That is how I designed it. I could have made this book three times as long, with more examples and references, but I do not believe this would be necessary to get my message across to you.

If you are new to wellness or if you are an experienced veteran, just know that wellness does not have to be complicated. You will soon find that it is easily grasped and can be smoothly integrated into your life.

A wellness lifestyle prevents the uncomfortable and promotes happiness. It is not intended to be an unpleasant chore. A strong wellness attitude and lifestyle is fun. It is fun to watch yourself mature. It is fun to smile all day long and to feel confident. It is fun not to have to go to the doctor's office and wait in lines for attention and for pills. It is fun to wake up each morning with an indescribable passion for life. It is fun to have enough energy to accomplish all your goals for the day. It is fun to have enough stamina to go on long hikes in nature. It is fun sharing wellness ideas with others. And finally, it is fun to give love freely.

Some people prefer to enter a swimming pool very slowly, one body/mind part at a time, and others prefer to run and jump in, head first. Either way is right. What I intend to reveal in this book, is that entering the wellness pool can take place for everyone at their own pace. Don't do it my way, do it your way! (But you still have to get your feet wet.)

I am in no way claiming to be a doctor, but I actually do follow the Hippocratic oath with the information I share in this book. Wellness follows the Hippocratic oath= Do no harm. Everyone is entitled to experience wellness! Reading this book will allow you to see what wellness is and how to invite wellness into your life forever.

Wellfully yours,
James Dennis

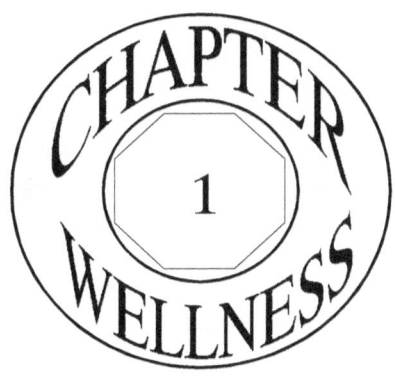

What is wellness?

Many definitions can be given. In fact, take a brief moment to state the first definition that comes to your mind/body.

The Webster's dictionary states that wellness is; *the quality or state of being in good health, especially as an actively sought goal*. This is a good definition, but for purposes that I will soon reveal, I have created a slightly modified version. The wellness definition I will be operating from in this presentation is; *an ongoing lifestyle in which a person chooses to develop their highest potential of health, happiness, and longevity*.

I realize this is a huge task to take on in one book, but I am up for the challenge. Are you? Great, lets do it then!

I will present a working model, which is my attempt to facilitate the understanding of wellness. It will give you something to visualize when the word, wellness, is used. I would like you to imagine an octagon.(That's a stop sign shape, in case you did not take geometry in school or managed somehow to avoid this class, as I did.) We will use the octagon to create eight areas of this wellness approach. I chose eight because it is a complete number with no beginning or end, and with good balance. Now imagine along the edge of each octagon line, there are these following words, which I will list alphabetically, as there is no one area that is more important than another:

Body/Mind, Career, Family/Friends, Fitness, Leisure, Nutrition, Sleep, and Spirituality.

These eight areas are the major components that make up all we do and are, in life. I could have divided wellness into twelve or one-hundred areas, however, this would terribly complicate matters, making it hard to digest or remember. And perhaps equally important, these eight areas are the ones that my intuition led me to, when I first created the Wellness For~Every~One concept. Furthermore, each area has subcategories, so anything you can think of can be placed in one of these eight areas, whichever area you feel it should go under. For instance, if you strongly feel that finances are a large part of wellness, you can place it under the category of career.

Now, in the middle of each border of the octagon, imagine a straight line extending out three inches or three feet, depending on how large you imagined your octagon to be. After doing this you will have an octagon with eight lines extending out from it. Next, I would like you to give yourself a grade on a scale of one to ten, for each separate wellness area. A number *one* represents that you feel you are doing poorly and you have many concerns in that area. A number *ten* means you feel you are doing excellent with no concerns in that area.

It is vital to give yourself the grade *you* feel is accurate, not the grade your doctor would give you or what your mom would give you. Simply state the number your first intuitive feeling gives, and mark it appropriately along the line, a ten being furthest away from the border. Do this quickly. All eight numbers should be filled out in less than one minute, to prevent over-analyzing. And do not worry about what each area's technical definition means, they are pretty self-explanatory, so just put down the number that corresponds to what you interpret each wellness area to represent. In the area of career, you may substitute school or volunteering in its place, if this is more appropriate. You are not bound by these numbers and only you will see them.

Now that you have completed this, connect all the dots.
{See the following example}

Wellness Rating Scale
1= poor / many concerns
10= excellent / no concerns

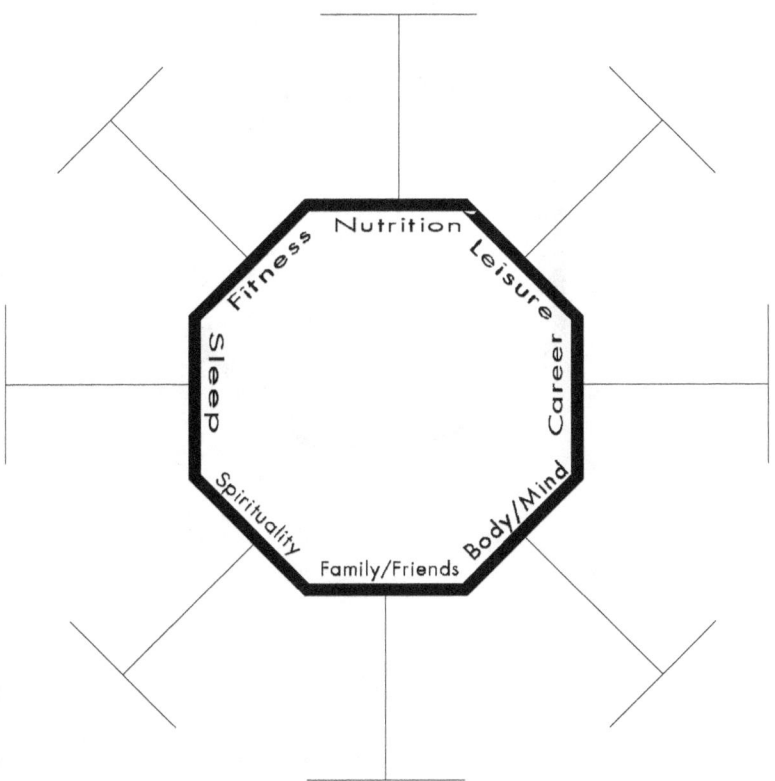

Make dashes appropriately along each line and then connect
the dots.

Example Diagram

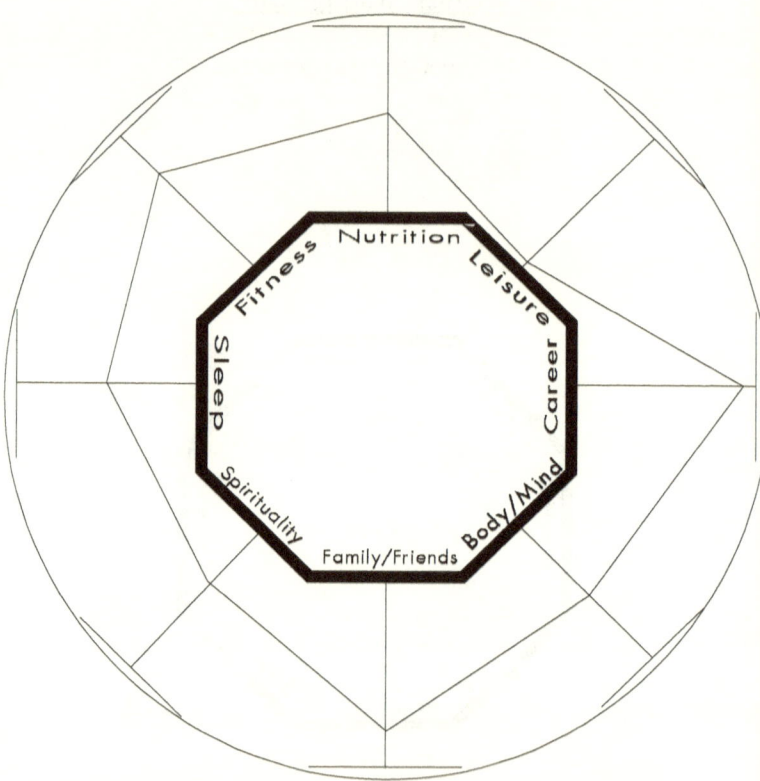

-The outside line represents a "complete" ten circle.
-The inside "perfect" shape is a generic wellness rating.

If you are like me, you might tend to skip over picking up a pencil and filling out this simple diagram. But please pick up the pencil this one time, which will only take one minute, and I promise you will not have to do any more physical labor while reading this book. Doing this is key, as we will refer to this diagram throughout the book.

We have all seen questionnaires in books and magazines that ask us to fill out lengthy multiple choice and true and false problems, and then you add up the points to see which category you fit in. Although I do not think doing this is a bad idea, I do not see many people filling them out. More importantly, the grade and category these tests put you under are not as important as the grade you give, the one you *feel* you deserve.(Try telling this to a high school student taking the SAT exam.)

One of the main purposes of this book is to place the responsibility of your wellness on you. The first step toward doing so requires you to give yourself a grade. After finishing this book, you will have the option of going back to the octagon model to change any rating, once you have the big picture of the unlimited possibilities wellness has to offer.

This octagon diagram allows you to see and remember what wellness represents, which is your whole life. Wellness does not only represent how many vitamins you should take or how many sit-ups you can perform, these are simply parts of wellness.

Connecting the Dots

Now that you have connected the dots, what does it look like? A square, an egg?

No, I am not going to diagnose you by what shape you have. This model simply gives us a good way to begin our exploration into wellness.

What would it have looked like if you answered 'ten' to everything? That's correct, a wheel or a circle! What is this the symbol for? Balance, flowing, the circle of life, and wholeness. Did you have a complete circle? I mean a complete-ten-circle, not a complete-two-circle? If you had a complete-ten-circle, thank you for joining me, there is no reason to stay any longer, so please give this book to a friend who is not so fortunate.

No wellness area takes priority over another, as they all equally support the whole-you. Certainly if you gave yourself a seven in all wellness areas except sleep, which is a score of two, it would make more sense to initially focus your attention on addressing sleep as soon as possible. But you do not need to sacrifice the strength of the other areas to improve your sleep.

Some people may argue that there is no complete-ten-circle. It may be difficult to conceive of a complete-ten-circle because;

1. Most of us have been taught that we are not now, and never will be good enough to be a perfect ten. Partly because we have been taught the "bigger and better" philosophy of life.
2. As we near ten, let's say you start off at a score of three in your sleep area, and you take steps which are working toward that perfect ten, over time your definition of what a ten represents has changed.

Why has it changed? As we learn, practice, and experience new possibilities, we realize what the **potential** of ten could bring.

Here is an Example: Sarah rates herself a three on the sleep scale because she wakes up often during the night, she snores, and she tosses and turns constantly. Sarah's idea of a ten sleep rating is only waking up once per night for no more than five minutes, to stop snoring after a hard day, and to toss and turn half as much. To her, initially, this is the definition of a ten or "heavenly sleep."

Now let's say, after four months of taking steps to reach her ideal sleep goal of ten, she has achieved all of her initial sleep goals, however, a ten in no longer a ten. Why?

Because she now realizes she would actually like to see herself sleeping eight hours a night, with no snoring at all, never waking up during the night, and she wants to remember at least one dream per night. And even then she has not reached a ten if her new goal is to master the art of lucid dreaming and out of body experiences. This could take forever.

So as you can see, our definition of superb sleep constantly changes as our knowledge and experience grows. This concept is true for all wellness areas.

Sometimes your wellness grade will improve without directly thinking about it. For instance, Tommy's body/mind and nutrition ratings were both a three, and he made many changes in his diet which have improved his nutrition score to a seven. Remarkably, his body/mind wellness rating has jumped to a six, even though he did not concentrate his efforts in this area at all. So improvements may be easier than you think, because all of the wellness areas support each other, sometimes in ways we never thought were related.

I used to think that spirituality had no relationship to my body/mind health, this was never even a remote consideration. The truth for me is that finding spirituality was my missing wellness area for many years, and I am constantly learning every day how this area allows me to fulfill the other seven areas.

A Perfect Ten

Having said all of this, I will now suggest:

Having a complete ten is not the main point! The main point is that we are moving in the right direction, toward ten and not zero.

Wellness is not some end point of ten that we reach after years of great trials.

The main thing I would like you to strongly consider, to know, and then practice is that your wellness circle is growing larger and larger, and not smaller and smaller. Obviously it is better to have a large wellness wheel as opposed to a small wheel. Because as we all know, when riding a bicycle, a large wheel goes further with less effort! It may be more challenging to get it started, but once it starts rolling, **watch out, you cannot stop it!!!**

Hopefully your wellness diagram looks more like a full circle as opposed to square or an egg, because a circle is more

7

balanced. And as many Eastern philosophies suggest, it is a lack of balance that prevents wellness. But first you have to be aware of what it is you are supposed to be balancing, which is the eight major wellness areas. A lack of balance may not only mean you are lacking in a certain area, it may mean you are spending excessive amounts of energy in a certain area. Exercise is important for wellness, but too much exercise can result in burn-out, injuries, and less time for the other seven areas.

I am not working off of the assumption that I know what everyone's wellness goals should be. We are all unique and therefore we will all have different ideas about what a complete wellness circle is supposed to be. And in the end, if life is going just the way you want it, then who am I or anyone else to tell you otherwise.

I have chosen to use the phrase "complete ten," and not "perfect ten," for a reason.

I will further attempt to confuse the issue by suggesting that whatever your wellness rating and shape is today, **is perfect now**!

"How can it be perfect if it is not a ten?" you ask in a puzzled manner.

It would depend on your definition of perfect.

Everything you have done up until this point in life has created your wellness rating today. Every choice you have made, every good fortune or misfortune that came your way, have all created the place you are at today. Nothing happens by accident. If it was supposed to happen another way, then it would have. If you were supposed to be rich and famous, then you would be. Can we agree on this? Therefore, your wellness score has to be perfect, what else could it be. Let me explain further.

What if we all operated off of the following premise:

We are all perfect exactly how we are!

"Well if we are all perfect, then why do we need this book or any other for that matter?" you demand.

Very good question.

I will propose a new concept, a paradigm shift, about this word, perfect. Who says you are not perfect? Your family, your friends, your boss. Guess what!, they do not have a say in this

8

matter.(Let he who is without sin--cast the first stone.) So forget about what anyone else tells you about your lack of perfection. You are the only one that needs to come to terms with the concept of your perfection. I mean really, wouldn't it be so much easier and more fun to operate from the knowing that you are perfect just the way you are now, the way you were yesterday, ten years ago, and tomorrow. If you are already perfect, then there is nothing to measure up to and there is no one you need to be better than. If you are perfect, then you no longer have to spend your time being a perfectionist. Instead of being a perfectionist, you can now spend your time being more spontaneous.

Just image this concept for a minute. To me it is simple because it is just a thought, just a belief, and I control my thoughts and beliefs.

"To believe this would be living a lie, it's a fantasy!" Joe Practical shouts.

To kindly borrow a phrase that Dr.Wayne Dyer often quotes, and one I often say to myself is: "You become what you think about all day long."

If you think you are not perfect now, never were and never will be, then that will be true, FOR YOU! But it's not true for me. So I will ask you to consider this paradigm shift, which is: **You are perfect right now, _and_ you choose to make changes which will lead to a greater experience of health, happiness and longevity.**

To some, this may seem to be a contradictory statement. We all change constantly, from birth to death, therefore it is not contradictory to make changes in the direction of wellness, and still remain perfect throughout. I would like to strongly suggest, if you have not already, to get a hold of the best selling _Conversations with God,_ by Neil Donald Walsch, to help you further understand this concept of perfection, and begin to incorporate it into your life.

The First Step Toward Wellness

Now that we have these wellness scores and concepts, what do we do with them?

You have two choices. You can say:

"OK, I am a rotten egg, and I like it that way, so what--we are all going to die anyway, see you later--have a nice life."

Or you can say:

"OK, I am a perfect egg, and I choose to develop my wellness wheel to get it rolling smoothly and on track, in order to fully experience optimal health, happiness and longevity."

Is one choice better than the other? **Absolutely not!** However, I will argue that the second choice will lead to greater joy, love, and freedom, and it is much more fun.

We all know people who would give the rotten egg response, and we know what kind of lifestyle they lead. It is their life, and they have every right not to strive for wellness. They are not bad people. They are simply *not ready* to begin this journey. I always emphasize the fact that some people are ready and some are not ready, no matter what the situation is. And maybe it will take several years, or perhaps lifetimes, before they are ready. So don't look down on these people. However, you may find more pleasure in life by not being in the company of these people. They are no better or worse than anyone. Just wish them luck, and be on your way.

Another common rotten egg response from the crowd will usually go something like, "We could be hit by a bus tomorrow, or the sky could fall any minute."

Yes, this is true, however, it is very unlikely. And basically that's what life is, playing the odds. What is the likelihood that anything we ever do will turn out the way we plan? My philosophy has always been to do the best I can to keep the odds in my favor. This is all I can do, and beyond that, it is out of my hands. Pessimists either believe that the odds are not in their favor, or they believe they do not deserve to have the odds in their favor.

A high level of wellness is not for a chosen few, we are all entitled to it. However, it does not come in a magic bullet.(At

10

least not yet.) Therefore, we have to decide how we want to *slide* along the 1-10 wellness scale.(Rather than climbing a ladder, which is too hard and scary, especially if you have acrophobia.) And now that you have made the choice to expand your wellness circle, as you glide along these paths, we should agree upon what tools are needed to get this "wellness ball" rolling.

Who gets to decide what wellness is? What qualifies as optimal health and happiness? How long is longevity anyway? The first tool we will utilize, the one that we already have available to us, which will help us decide what steps to take along our wellness journey, can be described as to use your; intuition, inner intelligence, innate intelligence, sixth sense, instinct, gut feeling, awareness, third eye, listening to yourself, rishi(which means the knower inside), or as OB-wan Kenobi said, "Use the force Luke."

All of these terms represent the same idea. You can choose any words you feel comfortable with. I will use all of these words interchangeably.

The above terms are commonly used concepts to be seriously explored. We hear them used every day, but are we taking full advantage of this gift, or do we usually push it out of the way and ignore it? Or do we think that these terms are mysterious, and if they were real, their presence would be written on stone tablets and fall from the sky? This may have been the way God spoke to Moses, but the odds are that your intuition will present itself in a more subtle fashion.

My favorite example of using your intuition is the story of the supposed wise man who was thought to be close to God. A terrible flood came suddenly to his town and he was forced to climb onto the roof of his house. He stood there calmly praying to God, to come and rescue him. Soon after he began to pray, a neighbor in row boat came by and offered to take him to safety. Surprisingly, the man simply said "No thank you, God is coming to save me." As he continued to pray, the sheriff zoomed by in large motor boat, yelling at the man to get in. But again the man sent the boat away stating, "My faith in God is very strong, he won't let me down." The water was quickly rising and was now up to his knees, when a helicopter flew over the roof and

11

dropped a rope to the man, pleading with him to grab on. But yet again, the man sent them away because his blind faith had convinced him that God was going to miraculously rescue him. Sadly the man drowned and soon went to heaven. The first question he asked God was,

"God, I prayed and prayed that you would come and save me from the flood, why didn't you answer my calls?"

God looked at him, opened his arms and whispered,

"Who do think sent the boats and the helicopter?"

Even if you have heard this story many times, I think it helps to drive home the idea of paying attention to your intuition. God/intuition is talking to you all the time, in all forms, as they are both omnipotent and omni-present. If the man was truly wise, he would have jumped in the first boat. That's what God/intuition is, it is the first boat!

I will now give a common example of how to use your awareness when making wellness decisions. I am not picking on smokers(however, they should be accustomed to it by now), but this is an easy way to illustrate how to use your intuition.

Will smoking lead to a positive development of my wellness? Not simply yes or no, but rather, what does my awareness tell me?

What does my nose tell me? Survey says, "Smells bad, burns my nostrils." (Initially this is easy to answer, however, if you have been smoking for a long time, your nose probably does not work anymore.)

What does my chest tell me? "Cough-cough, pain, go away."

What does my breath tell me? How about, "I'd rather eat raw garlic."(Which is great for you by the way.)

You get the picture, your intuition gave you the answer. This one was easy. Some decisions are not this easy. Not all questions you face will have such an obvious outcry from your intuition. One of the most challenging tasks I am asking you to undergo, is to allow your intuition to get involved, as if all wellness categories and habits are the first time you have ever encountered them. **You can do it!**

Your intuition is very smart and has a back up plan if you did not adhere to its first message. It's called trial and error,

12

cause and effect. You try smoking, and realize you are becoming addicted, you skip meals, your teeth get stained, etc. This is your intuition giving you another chance to see the light and remedy the situation.

We have yet another way to answer the question of whether a choice can lead to wellness, and that is by observing others. You do not have to ever experience the effects of smoking yourself to learn what the wellness choice is. You can see what habitual smoking does to the people around you. We are supposed to learn from others mistakes and successes. Can you imagine where we would be as a society if we all had to experience each mistake ourselves. We would still be living like cavemen/women.

The third method we will use to help choose our wellness path is to know what respectable studies tell us. For instance, almost every single study published on smoking reveals that it will kill us and does nothing for us in regard to wellness.

"Oh yea, what about George Burns, he smoked cigars every day, had a lot of girl- friends, and lived to his nineties."

George is not a good example because we know of his special relationship with God. Yes, these miracles do exist, but keep in mind, these people beat the odds. Did you ever consider that Mr. Burns could have lived to one-hundred-ten years old if he never smoked at all?

The fourth and final way to guide your wellness decisions, is to ask this important question: **"Is what I am doing now, benefiting me?"**

Why would you do anything in life that is not benefiting you? If it is not benefiting you, then what is preventing you from making a change?

Ideally, intuition, trial and error, the self-benefiting factor, and respectable studies will all come up with the same answers. But often it takes the researchers longer to come to sound conclusions, so stick with your intuition when in doubt.

Wrap Up

To finally wrap up this introduction, I would like to emphasize that you need to take responsibility for your actions, as I will advocate throughout this presentation. Blaming others is avoiding responsibility, and it cannot change the past or shape the future. No more blaming your upbringing, your genetic code, or God. From this day on, you will take full responsibility for making the choices that will lead you toward creating a bigger and brighter wellness wheel.

I am not so delusional to think that everything I do in regard to my wellness is the way for you. All I am delusional about is that my way works for me and your way can work for you, provided that we both develop an in-depth-lifetime relationship with our intuition. However, I am a passionate person with strong opinions, just like you, and I will let you know what they are throughout. Everything I suggest in this book is simple and sound. This information only contains unlimited beneficial possibilities and cannot harm you, because that is what wellness does, it prevents harm. And if it cannot harm you and may only help, then there is no excuse not to choose wellness.

We will now look at the eight wellness areas one by one. Let's start with nutrition, not that it is more important than any of the others, because I will routinely suggest that each area is important for complete wellness, to support each other, and to create good balance. If you have a wheel with missing spokes, yes it will roll for a while, but not smoothly and not for long. Consider this image when the ride of life gets a bit bumpy.

CHAPTER 2 NUTRITION

The common saying, "You are what you eat," sounds so simple and is yet extremely powerful. The more accurate phrase would read, "You are what you eat *and drink*."

We will first examine our liquid intake. Perhaps it is initially more important to understand this area, as we can live much longer on liquids alone, than food alone.

"What am I supposed to be drinking?" Remember to utilize the four tools mentioned in the last chapter, and always first ask yourself:

"What does my intuition tell me?" Your intuition recruits help from all of your senses, so use them.

"What do my eyes tell me?" Water is clear, natural, it falls from the sky, it flows from the rivers, and it ripples through the lakes. If God or the creator intended for us to drink coffee all day long, he would have created double mocha snow capped mountains and French Vanilla bunny slopes for us to ski down.

"What do my taste buds tell me?" Water goes down smooth at room temperature and it tastes good.

"What do my taste buds me about alcohol?" It burns as it goes down and it leaves a definite unpleasant smell on my breath.

"What do the studies tell me?" My body is mostly made of

15

water, not coffee or cola. We need water for blood filtration. Water helps the kidneys get rid of toxins, and it helps to move your bowels. Water is a vital component of every cell and cellular interaction in your body.

Sodas, processed-sugar-based fruit drinks, coffee, and alcohol are in a way the same. They all have additives, all are expensive, all can be addictive, and they are not a regular part of a wellness lifestyle.

The primary liquid I suggest is filtered water, such as from reverse osmosis or a high pressure carbon block filter, or any other method proven to be very pure with great taste. Stay away from tap water for drinking or cooking. Also, there are no regulations for the bottled water industry at this time, so check carefully on its source. Making water your main liquid is one of the easiest and most beneficial things you can do toward creating wellness. It is hard to drink too much of it, you cannot get drunk or hangovers from it (although plenty of water will help a hangover), you can't get sugar highs and lows from it, and you can't use it as an addictive excuse for not being able to start your day without it, as it is readily available. Simply go to the *well,* and reap the rewards.

Herbal teas and green tea can also be of benefit. Fresh juices, like from retail specialty juice stores or a juicer, are also terrific options. Yes it is better to actually eat the vegetable and fruit in its natural form, but the juice is still very good. I have yet to read any studies that suggest soda pop leads to longevity.

Alcohol

I do not need to give a lecture on the effects of alcohol. However, I cannot refrain from addressing this topic briefly. There are recent studies that suggest wine and other alcoholic beverages are good for the heart, and can lower cholesterol. To borrow a phrase from Dr. John McDougall, "People love to hear good things about their bad habits."

The truth is, alcohol makes the liver work overtime to rid toxins, it is a bladder irritant, it is addictive, and can often be the cause of deadly accidents. Alcohol dehydrates your body/mind.

Furthermore, studies show that alcohol kills brain cells. I don't know about you, but I need all the brain cells I can get.

Almost all of the wellness topics discussed only affect you directly. But in the case of drunk driving, your poor wellness habit can negatively change the lives of others. If you insist on reaping the possible benefits from alcohol, I suggest you get your hands on the original properties of alcohol, such as grapes, barely, or hops.

No good health practitioner would give sound advice to recommend that someone use alcohol regularly, as the risks far outweigh any possible benefits. I am not an extremist. I personally may have a sip of champagne at a wedding toast or holiday party, but I still don't like the taste.

Milk Box

It is now time for my one soap-box, or should I say milk-box.

Humans should only drink the milk of their mothers. Drinking cow's milk has got to be the most bizarre thing we could drink. And I was once as bizarre as millions of other wannabe cows, as my mother could barely keep enough milk in the refrigerator for her four kids. I did not like the taste of plain cow's milk, but I knew I was supposed to drink it to be big and strong, so I would mix in a large heaping of powdered chocolate to improve the taste.

I think it is ridiculous when studies come out every week that say, "Yes, it's true, breast feeding really is good for infants and mothers." What else could it be but perfect!

Mother Nature and sound studies simply reveal that breast milk is the only milk we need as infants. Mother Nature and studies also reveal that cow's milk is great, but only **for baby cows!!!** We also know that no other animal on earth drinks milk after it is weaned, as we are the only animal to out-smart our intuition in order to continue to drink milk into adulthood. Elephant milk is for elephants, and dog milk is for dogs. Have you ever seen a cow drink milk from a mother gorilla?

Cow's milk can be responsible for many illnesses, such as

ear infections, asthma, and auto-immune diseases, to name a few. I just read a study today, suggesting that schizophrenia and autism may have a relationship with the bodymind's inability to properly handle casein(a protein in cow's milk), which in turn produces chemicals that negatively affect the brain. No adult has ever been harmed by moving away from bovine milk.

If you are lactose intolerant, I have good news, there is nothing wrong with you. In fact, you should consider yourself lucky. Your bodymind is so smart that it screams at you to never drink cow's milk again. But some of us are smarter than our bodymind's intuition, and we take a special pill that tells the bodymind, "I know what does a body good, so haha, I can drink cow's milk if I want to."

I hope by now you realize that you absolutely do not need cow's milk to get your calcium. Calcium is not manifested by cows. Cows get calcium from the earth and so do you. In fact, a dietary deficiency in calcium and protein is unheard of, for the average person. Any doctor will admit to this.

Doctors and the dairy industry duped us into the notion many years ago, that cow's milk was better for kids than breast milk. I don't want to offend anyone for their past decisions, however, there is no excuse today. The greatest thing you can do for your newborn is to breast feed him/her until they are at least two years old. "If this is true, then why doesn't the American Medical Association say the same thing?" Well they do, in that the studies they publish promote breast milk. But you probably will not hear them tell you to never use cow's milk because of the many political ramifications that will result. (Remember the Oprah Winfrey-cattle farmer trial?)

Meals

How many meals should we eat each day? Most nutrition programs agree we should eat three or more meals a day, and smaller is better. This principle keeps metabolism up and keeps your intestines happy. If you ever had acid reflux or heart burn, this is your stomach yelling at you, "You ate too much of the wrong foods!" Indigestion, cramps, constipation, or loose stools, should not be happening on a regular basis. This is not normal. You do not get constipated because your body is deficient of laxatives.

The Ayervedic tradition suggests, and many European cultures practice, eating the largest meal at midday. And no plan suggests that dinner be your largest meal, especially not late at night. Studies suggest that a low caloric intake leads to longevity in animals. I have never seen photos of obese centenarians on television with Willard Scott, have you?

The more we eat, the more we have to work to get rid of the excess. The overweight population not only suffers from eating the wrong foods, but too much of it. And if you are someone who considers yourself lucky because you can eat any and everything and not gain weight, does not mean you are on a wellness path. In fact, I might suggest that overweight people are lucky. At least they can see there is a problem that needs to be dealt with. Thin people have heart and brain attacks just like obese people do.

Our evolution is partly responsible for our tendency to over eat when food is available, to prepare for times when food might not be available. However, a lack of available food is not a problem for most people in industrialized societies.

If you ate five smaller meals and plenty of water each day, you probably would not feel the urge to consume large amounts of food. Instead of having seconds, save it for the next meal. If you cannot get past the adage that you have to clean your plate, then get a smaller plate and a smaller fork.

Slow Down

Have you ever eaten at a restaurant with a friend, and you order the same meal. You both start to eat at the same time but one of you finishes fifteen minutes before the other? A good general principle is to slow down when you eat. Did you ever hear your mother say "Eat faster kid it's good for you?" Biting your tongue or lip during mealtime is your sixth sense blatantly shouting at you to "Slow down already, eating is not a race." Put your fork down after each bite, the food is not going anywhere.

Eat every bite as if it were your last bite on earth. If you are contemplating eating more food after your first modest serving, wait for five minutes before you reach for more. You may amazingly find that once your satiation hormones have a chance to assess the amount of food in your stomach, you may not decide to fill your plate again.

Try this simple experiment to help you slow down during meals:

The second after you put a piece of food into your mouth, close your eyes and keep them closed until the next bite. Maintain all of your attention on the food. Notice how it tastes, how it smells, what the texture is like, what it feels like as you swallow. If your thoughts wander, simply bring them back to the food. Do this for the entire meal and reflect on its effect on you.

This amazing exercise heightens your awareness to the joys of eating, and can actually be considered a form of meditation.

It is difficult to meditate with the television on, so turn the television off. Why would you want to look at tragic death scenes during dinner? A novel idea would be to talk to those in your company, while playing soft music in the background.

Be grateful for each meal. Thank the chef at the restaurant personally, they love to hear it. And do not forget to thank the household chef for **every** meal they cook, regardless of the taste.

The Right Diet?

Eating is one of the greatest joys in life! It is also personal and sacred. There are so many diet programs, cookbooks, and television shows that all have different views. How can they all be correct? How is one to decide?

The first question to ask is, "Is the way I am eating now, providing what I want, and is it leading me along the wellness path?"

What do your eyes tell you?

Is it that food should be colorful and pleasing to look at? Do you like the looks of a bright green kiwi and a shiny orange, or do your eyes prefer the looks of a gray bloody hamburger or an off white piece of pork? Honestly, what *looks* better?

What smells better, a fresh baked home-made apple pie, or a pot of boiling chicken?

What would your hands rather hold, a ripe tomato, or an uncooked slimy drumstick?

What does your intuition tell you, **not, what do the fast food commercials tell you!**

I would like to now recommend a best selling book titled *Diet for a New America*, by John Robbins. It is very easy to get your hands on this information, in order to *truly* heighten your awareness of food/nutrition. I am not stating to necessarily follow his diet recommendations, which by the way can be very beneficial for some. He looks at this subject from, in my opinion, an enlightened point of view.

There is so much varying information out there right now, however, most reputable experts agree to decrease saturated fat and animal products, and to increase fruits and vegetables. It is reasonable to say that we are all unique and therefore we all have unique nutritional needs, that may change over a lifetime. So for me or anyone to suggest that we all eat exactly the same, is not realistic. All studies are basically reporting the same themes. **None** of the studies are suggesting to eat more Double Whoppers with Cheese or to stay away from fruits and vegetables.

If your current ethnic foods are nutritiously limiting, consider expanding your comfort zone. In San Francisco there are so many places to eat, you could try a new restaurant every day for several years and you still wouldn't have tried them all. How about being spontaneous the next time you eat out, and expose yourself to a new healthy ethnic dish. Spontaneity is your intuition wanting you to experience life to its fullest, and eating is a very safe way to explore this spontaneity.

Eating should be fun and simple. I do not believe it was meant to be complicated, like counting every calorie and weighing your foods. A simple rule I am now following is to make sure I have at least one fresh fruit or vegetable with each meal. French fries with ketchup and pickles do not count.

Snacks and Desserts

Many things we consider to be snacks are highly processed and prepackaged. However, if you ate five small meals a day you wouldn't have much of a need for snacks. If you have a craving for a snack, choose a piece of fruit, not a cupcake! Fruits can be fantastic desserts as well. Cheesecake is not part of a wellness lifestyle. Now like I said, I am not an extremist, perhaps once a year, **but not every week.**

If you crave something sweet, I honestly believe that fruit will serve the purpose if you give it a chance. On the other hand, I also believe that it's not good to totally deny yourself of your favorite rich treat. But when do you draw the line: once a day, once a week, one bite, two, three...? I always say that the second and third bite of a rich chocolate mousse usually tastes just as good as the first. So just have the first bite and experience this moment of pleasure and move on.

Lately, it seems the buzz word in the area of nutrition is "moderation." In general, I agree with this recommendation, however, the term moderation can be vague. If a man eats at a fast food restaurant seven days a week, eating these foods only four times a week could be considered moderation for his usual practices. If a woman never eats fresh fruits, she may assume that moderation means eating fresh fruit three times a week instead of three times a day. So don't fool your inner self with misconceptions about the term "moderation."

In the end, you are responsible for buying your foods. If you do not buy double stuffed-cream filled cookies or high fat ice creams, it makes it hard to consume them at home. If you don't know how to prepare "good for you" foods, that's OK, there are literally hundreds of cookbooks available. Or better still, find a nutrition mentor. I have yet to meet a person that does not like to share their favorite healthy recipe. And if you are someone who tries to convince yourself that you cannot eat healthier because you are a terrible cook, just remember, you become what you think about all day long.

Nutrients

What about supplements? I suggest that we all should take a multi-vitamin/mineral supplement at the very least. (Unless you are someone like Gary Null, the super-nutrition-man.) They cost pennies a day and can only help you, some more than others, and they are safe. Our soils have become scarce of some nutrients, so we may not be getting them all through our foods. Many illnesses can be directly related to a deficiency of vitamins and minerals. Numerous books and internet sites are good resources to find out how illnesses can be helped by specific vitamins, minerals, and herbs. Go to the internet and check out: **www.Drweil.com**, and fill out a simple questionnaire to get specific supplement recommendations. This is the only web site I will recommend in this book as a wellness resource, so use it-- you will not be disappointed.

Using supplements does not give you an excuse for skipping meals or eating unbalanced meals. I do strongly suggest that you consider modifying your diet as a means to addressing various discomforts, as opposed to always paying big bucks for doctors and pills. For instance, eliminating all caffeine and chocolate from your diet may cure you of the migraine headaches you have been getting for years. The list of relationships between nutrient to illness, literally goes on and on.

Most all nutrition programs say to eat more carbohydrates than protein and fat. But what are the right percentages? I think high carbohydrates are fine if they are not from candy, flour, alcohol, or soda. Instead, we should consume complex carbohydrates like whole grains, fruits, vegetables, beans, and brown rice. Excess protein leaches calcium from your bones and can lead to osteoporosis and kidney damage.

If we consider breast milk to be a perfect food, and less than six percent of its calories are from protein, and this is the greatest time in life when we need protein for growth, then why would we need high percentages of protein as adults? Most people in affluent societies experience problems from excess protein and not a lack of it. If you were lacking protein, your hair and finger nails would not grow and a simple paper cut would not heal.

It is harder to get fat if you do not eat fat. There is fat in most all foods, so we do not need it from unnatural sources like margarine or vegetable shortening.(See chapter ten on "change," to help you make new food choices.) I only use extra virgin olive oil minimally for cooking as it is the most beneficial form of fat that studies point to.

If your eating habits are not benefiting you now, they never will. Going on a new diet to lose weight makes no sense if your intention is to eventually go back to eating the same way as you did before the weight loss. If your intuition and nutritional studies do not show you the way, trial and error will most certainly reveal the right formula. The challenge is to make the effort to stick with the trails long enough to see if any errors occur. Trying a new diet for one day probably will not prove highly effective. Instead, stick to the new diet for at least one month, before you decide if it is benefiting you or not. Whichever diet you choose, I hope you would be happy with the choice, and that your intention would be to maintain this working formula on a long-term basis.

I could talk about nutrition all day, however, I feel there is plenty of information out there to further help you along this path, and the truth is that you have all the tools you need already. Finally, I will reiterate that nutrition is a vital component of wellness and affects your performance in all other wellness categories. One area that nutrition can support is the wellness area of sleep. So now onto one of my favorite things to do, sleep.

CHAPTER 3 SLEEP

Sleep is another great joy in life. When I hear someone say, "I never sleep, I haven't had a good night rest in months," I wonder, how can this be? But indeed, for some this is an all-to-real situation. I have seen what a lack of sleep for several nights can do to a person, with my own eyes. It is very scary! There are many areas that can be examined to find out what is preventing a good night sleep.

What hours do you sleep? Are they regular? Do they change daily or on weekends?

It is important to establish a consistent sleep time. This includes your days off work.

Personally, I sleep between 9-10 PM and wake up around 6-7 AM, which is at least eight hours but rarely more or less. This is how my biological clock works, it has always been that way.

We are all influenced by our circadian rhythm, which is an internal clock that tells us when we should be asleep and awake. I would like to refer you to *Sleep Thieves,* a book by Stanley Coren. He is a very fun author, whom you should enjoy. In the book he points out how Thomas Edison's invention of the light bulb altered the human species' evolution instantly. Before the light bulb, we all presumably went to sleep when it got dark and woke up when the sun came up. So the light bulb has confused our circadian rhythm and thrown us off balance.

Should we ask our old friend, our third eye, which sleep path will lead to wellness? Should we deny thousands of years of evolution? Or should we give into the notion that it is too late, and that we cannot undo the light bulb?

Up all Night

I learned about my circadian rhythm and the effects of denying evolution, the hard way. When I was eighteen years old, I took a job for the United Parcel Service(UPS). I felt I was strong enough for this work, and the pay was handsome for an eighteen-year-old, plus benefits. The only catch was that I had to start work at 3:30 AM. "No problem," I thought. "I will just go to bed a few hours early to make up for the lost morning hours." To make a short story shorter, I quit after three days. I did not care if the pay was doubled and the work was cut in half. I felt horrible and sick to my stomach, with giant headaches, which I never get. I listened to my intuition and swore to never do anything to jeopardize my wellness sleep area again.

Another message from my inner awareness, helped me cruise through school. I can vividly remember one night, three friends and I were studying the eve of an important Occupational Therapy exam. We studied from 7-9 PM, and then I stood up, yawned and said, "We've made some good progress tonight, now it's time to go home and get some sleep."

They laughed, and thought I was joking. And I thought they were joking when they replied, "We are just getting started, who's going to make the next pot of coffee?"

I have never pulled an all night cram session. I always felt I would be better-off getting plenty of sleep. At least then I would feel sharp enough to come up with a creative answer, and I would be more able to access my long term memory. This always worked better, as opposed to temporarily memorizing bits of information that I would probably soon forget after the test. And all night cramming is not necessary if you do not procrastinate, which I never did.

How Long is Enough

What if you only sleep five hours a day, you have plenty of energy, feel well rested, and your life is great? What if your body/mind does not let you sleep more than five hours, assuming the sleep conditions were optimal for longer rest? The answer would have to be, if your intuition tells you that you are sleeping fine, then by God, there is no problem. Many people I know would love to only sleep a few hours a night, and still be full of energy and clarity. This would allow them to do more things during the day. But I think this is the exception and not the norm.

Sleeping-in does not help, meaning, you fully awaken at 6 AM, but you do not get out of bed until 10 AM, because you are trying to catch up on lost sleep from the past three rocky nights. The bad news is that studies show this does not work and will actually cause you to have less energy the day. So don't just lie there staring at the ceiling, get out of bed! Mr.Coren's book shows that we were designed to sleep nine to ten hours a day, and preventing this from occurring will increase the likelihood of accidents and mistakes, some life threatening. For example, if a doctor, truck driver, or airline pilot are in a sleep debt, the results could be and have been, deadly.

How do you know if you are getting enough sleep? One obvious answer your innate intelligence plainly gives, is that if you need an alarm clock to wake you up every day, then you are not getting enough sleep. If you would rather stay in bed during an earthquake instead of crawling to a safe place, you need more sleep. If your ex-wife comes barreling into your room, screaming that you just won the lottery, and you mumble, "That's nice dear, you can have it, now go away," you need more sleep.

Even a subtle loss of sleep can result in things like increased irritability, decreased attention span, mood changes, and delayed reaction time. Which all scare me, especially in regard to other drivers on the road.

Everyone at work knows if you didn't get enough sleep, it's written all over your face. And if they cannot read your face, you are sure to tell them how poorly you slept and how not to expect too much from you today. You can also read the face of a person who works swing shifts, because humans were not built to work swing shifts.

Can you imagine what people would be like in a city that never sleeps? Some of you may be night owls and you cannot imagine going to sleep before midnight. You probably did not always do this, especially when you were a kid, but for some reason you changed. Therefore, if you are a night owl, it would not make sense to have a job that requires you to start at 7 AM. Wouldn't it make more sense to know your unique circadian rhythm and schedule your lifestyle accordingly? For instance, I have not made a New Years Eve midnight in many years. This is not because I am a party pooper, but it is extremely difficult for me to stay up that late. I don't fight the clock, I use it in my favor. I am one of these guys who night owls hoot at, as I like to exercise early in the morning.

Erase the notion from your mind that sleeping too much is a sign of being a lazy bum. No more guilt about sleeping more than the average guy. If the respectable studies, your intuition, and trial and error are telling you to get more sleep, then why are you not listening! Take just one week to arrange your schedule so it allows for consistent uninterrupted sleep. Then take an honest evaluation of how doing this affected your performance and happiness throughout the week. The benefits could be surprising.

Highs and Lows

It is interesting to know that our circadian rhythm has low points that we should be aware of. Between 1-4 AM and 1-4 PM, we are more sleepy than at other times of the day. Just try waking someone up at 2 o'clock AM and see how long it takes for them to come about. And I think we all know the feeling we get after lunch, and how we wouldn't mind taking a quick nap at 2 PM, if the boss wasn't around. We also have spikes in our circadian rhythms at 9-11 AM and 7-9 PM, when we are more likely to have clarity and energy, regardless of the amount of sleep we had the night before.

I think it is beneficial to be aware of these cycles. I may be more likely to make various plans, using these facts in my favor. For instance, I would want to schedule a job interview for 10 o'clock AM, when I will look and feel sharp and enthusiastic. And hopefully the interviewer will also be awake, and will actually remember who I was and what I said, when it is time to make the hiring decisions. If I were a CEO, I would not schedule the most important meeting of the year at 2:30 PM, because my employees would be sleeping in the back of the room.

Environment

Your environment plays a huge part of a restful slumber. Temperature is a definite key.

Have you ever tried to sleep during the hottest night of the summer? **Forget about it.** It is actually better to have the environment be a little bit cooler, than hotter. Consider giving away your electric blanket. It may actually be harmful because of the electro-magnetic field it creates. Also, our body temperature drops a few degrees when we sleep, so tough it out for a minute when you crawl into a not so warm bed tonight, you may fall asleep easier. Make sure you have enough blankets to prevent waking up and feeling cold in the middle of the night. And if you know who keeps kicking off my wife's side of the blankets during the night, would you ask him if he would stop doing this if I put less blankets on in the first place?

Outside noises need to be eliminated, this is obvious. There is a device called a white noise generator that you can use in your room to drown out various noises, to help you stay sleep. Other devices like a fan, air conditioner, or air vents provide similar effects. Also, try playing your favorite deep-relaxing compact disc, and put it on repeat, all night long. It can't hurt to try. You might also consider new sound proof windows, for when the garbage man comes around. Finally, thick curtains or shades will prevent early morning sun light from entering the room and waking up night owls too early.

I would like to point you in the direction of the ancient Chinese art of "Feng Shui." This subject deals strictly with creating the optimum environment, not only for your bedroom, but for your entire house and workplace. Some things Feng Shui teachers suggest in the bedroom is that you should be able to see the bedroom door and all windows from where you sleep. They also suggest to keep nothing between your bed and the floor.(Like to store your "stuff".) Keep bathroom doors closed and have plants in each room. A large part of this art, is utilizing compass directions and various colors and shapes around the room to promote comfort. These suggestions can even promote a more passionate love life. Feng Shui is actually very interesting and I have had good results from these suggestions.

Equally effective recommendations would be to use therapeutic pillows for anyone having trouble sleeping or waking up with a stiff neck. These pillows cradle your neck in a natural position, and it is a very wise investment. Experiment with different ways of positioning yourself with pillows, like a body pillow. Also, I hear advertisements daily about retail specialty stores where you can get a new mattress, money-back guaranteed for ninety days with free delivery. You have nothing to lose and everything to gain from trying a new mattress.

Still Can't Sleep

A total lack of sleep for more than two days is very serious and needs to be addressed today. There are very effective herbal remedies that are safe and can help you fall asleep, such as valerian, passion flower, and hops. You can use these aids occasionally, but you should not have to rely on sleeping pills, Nyquil, or herbal teas every night to go to sleep.

A hot bath before bedtime is a natural and powerful method to put you to sleep, and of course, feels great and relaxes you. Other tips to fall asleep are to read a book, watch television (something other than violence or the late night news), or listen to relaxing music. All three interventions slow down your brain waves, which is what your brain does when you sleep. Also, keep a sleep journal to help you see what may be contributing to irregular sleep, such as late night snacking or inconsistent sleep times. Try all of these safe methods before dragging yourself to the doctor, begging her for some sleeping pills.

If you or your partner snore, you may joke about it with them, however, they could be experiencing sleep apnea, which is a life threatening condition. In Stanley Coren's book he told about a sleep study they did on a man who snored, and was not functioning well in the daytime. He actually woke up 456 times during the night because of this condition. The man only thought he woke up six times that night. The truth is, he never reached the deep part of sleep that we are all supposed to have at night. He was really experiencing the feeling you get when you are just about to fall asleep, but each time his need for more oxygen would result in a jarring snore, preventing normal sleep.

Sleep apnea and snoring can definitely be improved through losing weight, eliminating alcohol and tobacco, and sleeping on your side or stomach, instead of your back.

We have all had the experience of having our thoughts race **all over** the place at night, worrying about "this and that," praying to God and the sandman to let us fall asleep already. At least then we could let our dreams worry about "this and that," while we get some rest. Instead of tossing and turning for three hours, go out of the room and read a book until you become sleepy again.(Or you may try convincing your significant other that you need an emergency orgasm in the middle of the night, if this helps you fall asleep quickly.) I will discuss our thought processes when we get to the body/mind wellness area, to offer more assistance with this problem.

What about when your baby wakes up in the middle of the night, crying for food?

I can speak first hand about how to handle this.(Sleep with ear plugs.) No, just kidding.

My baby would sleep in her crib at the beginning of the night, so Dori and I could at least have some cuddle time. In the middle of the night, when Noelani woke up, Dori or I would pick her up and bring her to our bed, which was in the same room. Dori would lift up her shirt to feed Noe, while lying in bed, half asleep. Noelani would get her tummy full and quickly fall back to sleep, remaining the rest of the night in bed with us. And Dori was so exhausted(as she also was working and going to school)she would fall right back to sleep. Many times I was none the wiser. We did this for two years.

We did not have to heat milk, rock her to sleep, or deal with colic. Intuition and cause and effect told us it was the right thing to do for restful sleep, for all three of us. This was very simple and it worked. By the way, Noe only had colic one time as an infant, and it was coincidentally when Dori drank cow's milk during the day, which she had not done up until that point of nursing, which probably was passed along to Noe. Dori never drank cow's milk again, while breast feeding, and Noe never got colic again. Even today, Noelani sleeps from around 9 PM to7 AM, and does not wake us up in the middle of the night. And she rarely takes naps, although it would be nice if she did.

Dreams

Dreams are very beneficial, they serve a purpose and they are necessary. One way to think about dreams, is that it may be an avenue for your soul to leave your body, to be free. One possibility is; what if every time you dreamt, let's say about you and a friend at the movies, that both of your souls were actually meeting on a different astral-plane? Possibly, but what about when your friend doesn't have the same dream that night? Maybe your friend did, and simply did not remember it! Honestly, do you always contact each person you dream about, the next morning, to see if they had the same dream? Anyway, I think this is a fun way to look at my dreams. It makes them so much more real. It is also a bunch of fun sharing dreams with others and figuring out what they might mean.

Everyone dreams during sleep, and don't forget about daydreaming. If you are someone who says you cannot remember anything about your dreams, there is hope. I would encourage you to learn about dream states, such as "out of body experiences" and "lucid dreaming." There are numerous book titles that teach how to do this and how to interpret dreams. I have been keeping a pad and pencil on my night-stand, so I can blindly jot down keywords in the night, about my dreams, in order to spark my memory of them the next morning. This does not interfere with my sleep, and it seems like all of a sudden, I am accessing my dreams more than I ever have before. It is fun and amazing to realize how much I dream each night.

I would now like to point you in the direction of "Dreamland," a Sunday night radio talk-show, hosted by Art Bell. This show will provide you with many dream enhancing resources.

"Oh no" you say, "Not the UFO guy." Please do not tune me out yet.

Mr. Bell has created a forum for the unknown, the difficult to explain. He is a skeptic in a lot of regards. Initially, I thought this show was crazy. All I can say is to give it a chance. He frequently has on guests that are doctors, Ph.D.s, cardinals, movie directors, and NASA scientists. They are usually very respected professionals in their fields. O.K., so once in a while he has on a guy who claims to be a vampire, but you can turn it off and try again next week, if you want. He is also on the radio for five hours during the weeknights, nationwide, and on the internet. So if you can't go back to sleep one night, listen for a while and learn something, and at the least, you will be entertained.

I would like to recommend a movie called *What Dreams May Come,* which you may have already seen. I don't know about you, but this movie moved me deeply. I can't say enough good things about it. (One area the movie focused on was suicide. I don't necessarily buy into the writer's explanation of what happens to those who take their own life, but I do think that if all people considering suicide could see this film, they would be scared silly, and would try everything possible to work out their problems here on earth.)

If none of the above suggestions do the trick to obtain sound sleep and vivid dreams, I would not hesitate to refer you to a hypnotist. There is no reason to be afraid of hypnosis. It cannot harm you, when conducted by an experienced therapist. Hypnosis may allow you to find out what is truly preventing restful sleep. A nice introduction into the benefits of hypnosis is a book titled *Soul Healing*, by Bruce Goldberg. In this book he attributes the healing of various bodymind illnesses to hypnosis. If anything, hypnosis will help you to relax and to remember important events.

Sleep should be easy and fun. I would hope it is, because for many of us it consists of 1/3 of our lifetime. Sleep is a time for the mind/body to grow and recuperate. Sleep is an absolute key factor for experiencing a high level of wellness. Moving in the right direction along this wellness path may produce new happiness you never dreamt possible. And some say that dreaming is the souls way of getting closer to spirituality. Let's now explore this topic in the next chapter.

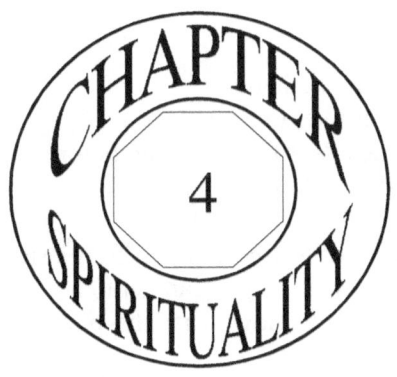

CHAPTER 4 SPIRITUALITY

What does spirituality have to do with wellness?

I will ask for your open bodyminded attention as we enter the realm of spirituality. I am not going to try to convert you into anything, so just simply have some fun, as I pose the most famous question of all time.

What is the meaning/purpose of life?

Please take a moment to state your answer to this aloud.

This may sound like a question for the philosophers, but it is hard to talk about spirituality without talking about philosophy. I will bet there are many of you who have never come up with a stated answer to this question, although we have all thought about it in some form at some time. How long did it take to create or remember, an answer? Was your definition clear and succinct? If you do not have your own explanation of life's purpose/meaning, make it a priority to come up with one. Your explanation could be influenced by your religious leader, a book, you can ask a friend, or meditate on it.

If there is any definition you ever know by heart, I will argue that your definition of what the meaning/purpose of life is, should come to you as easy like a Sunday morning.

I do want to be very clear that I am not saying there is necessarily a universally correct answer, or that you should follow my purpose of life. I advocate self exploration, because:

The purpose/meaning of life can be whatever we want it to be!

It could be:

-To live fast and die hard.

-To live and let live, live and let die.

-To get as much "stuff" as you can before you go.

-To have children, to reproduce.

It could be:

-To suffer pain, or to free yourself from original sin.

-To serve your God, so you can get to heaven.

-Whatever, I don't know what the purpose of life is and I don't care.

-There is no purpose of life (This belief makes it too easy to commit suicide.)

It could be one of a million definitions.

Many great philosophers have written on this subject, as humans have been pondering this question for many moons. I am not a Tibetan Buddhist, nor do I know too much about Buddhism. However, I am interested in all forms of spirituality, and I recently read a book called *The Art of Happiness*, by Howard Cutler M.D. In this book, he presents material gathered from his relationship with the Dalai Lama. It was unique, in that, Mr.Cutler allows his reader to understand Buddhism from a Western culture- dogmatic viewpoint.

I was immediately consumed by the Dalai Lama's basic premise of living. The Dalai Lama states, **"The purpose of life is happiness."** This is not a profound statement, but powerful nonetheless. Let us now follow this notion for a moment, and see how it relates to expanding wellness.

If we make the core reason for living, to experience happiness, then our wellness decisions will be much easier to make. My previous answer to the purpose of life, I learned in a summer philosophy class. Before that class, I do not remember having an explanation nor did I ever have someone ask me what I thought the meaning of life was. My former belief was that we are here to learn as much as we can, and then we are to share our knowledge with others. This would help to expand a higher level of knowledge so the human race could progress to bigger and better things. However, through the Dalai Lama's simple teaching, my core foundational belief is now that, *the purpose of life is happiness*.

Why is this significant? If I base all my choices on this premise, then answers to my questions will always lead me down the right path, where else could it take me!

Allow me to explain. Going back to my previous purpose of life, I would try to learn as much as possible so I could then share this knowledge with others. In a lot of ways this is a good thing, but it does not necessarily lead to my happiness. Learning and helping others can lead to happiness and pleasure, but my focus was not necessarily on my happiness, as it was, to gain pleasure from seeing others improve from my teachings. I would read material and think, "How can I use this information to help others?" instead of focusing on the here and now. An even better question to ask would be, "How can this information better me and how can it contribute to my own happiness?"

To strive for ones own happiness is not selfish. If you are truly a happy person inside and out, then that is what people will see in you, they will feed off it. Hopefully they will then share this happiness with others, and so on and so on. I am not suggesting that you attain happiness at the cost of causing undue harm to others, this would not bring good karma.

Is this sort of clear so far?

If we make the premise of life--to experience happiness, I don't see how we can go wrong. I am now making this shift. I am regularly catching myself doing novel things and the first thought is, "How can I use this experience to help my clients?" And then I will say, "Whoa, wait a minute Jim, come back to the here and now, and experience how this affects your happiness and well-being. When the time is right, you will be able to appropriately share this information with others." This shift will take practice, maybe months or years, but that's fine. Each time it will get easier.

There is then the logical question that follows, which I am sure you have already thought of, which is, "What is happiness?"

I suppose you are the only one who can answer this question.

Maybe happiness is innate and we all know the answer deep down, we just have to look within ourselves.

In order to fully understand happiness, we have to distinguish between happiness and pleasure. Certainly they can be the same thing. And in addition to this, we have to distinguish between happiness and avoiding pain.

Eating an eclair every day is very pleasurable for most, myself included. And why shouldn't we experience pleasure, it feels great. Well, the question is, do you want pleasure or do you want happiness? Is happiness looking and feeling fit, and being full of energy with clean arteries, or is happiness an eclair?

Eating a ripe strawberry may create great pleasure for your taste buds and will also create happiness because it has many favorable nutritional properties, leading you along your nutritional wellness path. We can also use this strawberry for an example of avoiding pain. Maybe you think you are happy by eating a strawberry, but are you actually avoiding the pain associated with eating your favorite high fat-strawberry ice cream, because you cannot stand to put on another pound. You are not eating the strawberry for the pleasure or happiness it brings, you are eating it because you hate the pains of being obese.

Let me give another example of how this happiness theme plays out. What should I do if my child is doing something I feel needs disciplining, like hitting the dog for no reason? Disciplining my child does not bring me pleasure, and in fact, it may even be painful. However, knowing that this brief moment of discipline proves to lead toward long term happiness(at least for the dog), I know I am making the right choice for family wellness.

Now let's pick a super difficult question. Let's say Sam is contemplating being unfaithful to his spouse. The opportunity is right there before him, and all he can think about is the pleasure he is in store for. Or maybe all he can think about is dulling the pain from a recent hurtful argument with his spouse.

If Sam's basic meaning of life is happiness, and if he asks himself the question, "Will this act of adultery lead to happiness?" then the decision should be much easier. If his relationship with his spouse is making him happy in general, has been mostly happy in the past, and promises to be happy in the future, and knowing that if he made a decision to go with pleasure or to avoid pain, he would certainly jeopardize this happiness, then he knows that the answer is to walk away.

"What if giving into pleasure or dulling pain, now, will lead to greater happiness down the road?"

Only you can answer this. If you and your intuition truly-100% believe that you should cheat on your spouse because it will lead to happiness, then do it. (In most cases it won't.)

I can just see the ladies in the audience shaking their fingers at me right now saying, "How could you suggest that, what about the family, it could be broken up."

Again, if Sam sacrifices his happiness and turns away from his basic premise of life's purpose, then he is going to be miserable. Should Sam stay in this relationship for years and make everyone else unhappy, which may lead to other problems? Again, I chose one of the most complicated examples, but I hope you can see my point.

I recently asked my wife what she thought the purpose of life was. She said it was "To have children." This made sense because she does love children, and she is studying to be a grammar school teacher. I suggested that this purpose of life could be problematic because she will not have children forever, and may not have kids for a long time or ever again. Her belief of achieving happiness--revolves around her ability to successfully reproduce. She agreed, and has modified her meaning of life, which is, "To *care* for children."

Operating from this new purpose of life, she can now make better wellness choices. She knows that exercising regularly will increase her odds of staying fit enough to raise our daughter and to teach her students. Eating a balanced diet will lead to increased energy and health which will provide for more child rearing experiences. Not exercising at all and eating junk foods would impair her ability to carry out her stated purpose of life.

I remain convinced that we need to come up with a stated reason for living. You do not necessarily have to follow the Dalai Lama(although he has lived fourteen lifetimes, he must know something), and certainly he is not the only one who suggests this happiness theme. Maybe you already believed this on your own, good for you. But in the end, you have to come up with something, because this will surely affect your wellness.

What does all of this happiness business have to do with spirituality?

I believe the easiest and most natural way to find God-your spirituality is through happiness. I do not believe we are here on earth to experience unhappiness, because I am an optimist and not a fatalist. Living in a state of happiness benefits me. Living in a state of unhappiness does not benefit me. And it is arguably extremely difficult to find your spiritual nature while in a state of unhappiness.

I am sure that everyone would agree that miracles are happy events. And aren't miracles sent by God? As Albert Einstein said, "There are two ways to look at life. One is as though nothing is a miracle. The other is as though *everything* is a miracle."

Incorporating the knowing that everything is a miracle and not merely a coincidence, into your life, will expose your spirituality to you and to everyone that comes into contact with you.

I had to create *my own* beliefs about how God could benefit me. That is the fun part of spirituality, you can create any belief you want, because there is no wrong answer. The only right answer, is right, if it works for you and brings happiness. And I can modify my beliefs throughout life as I learn more and more about my spirituality.

Religion

I would like to differentiate between religion and spirituality, because many think that they are the same thing. Religions are created by people, a group of people who follow the same practices. Catholics, Muslims and the Jewish are common examples. Spirituality was created by God, and has been around long before religion. You are born with a spirit/soul, but you were not necessarily born with a religion.

40

The quote you may be familiar with is that, "We are all *spiritual* beings having a human experience." The saying is not that we are all *religious* beings having a human experience. Please do not get me wrong, I respect all religions, and I think they can provide tremendous benefits to many people. I have seen these benefits with my own eyes. We have seen mass destruction in the name of religion, as well. The word spirituality is always inclusive, but religion is not always inclusive. Religions come and go, but spirituality is eternal. Spirituality is *your* relationship with God/the world, not your religion's relationship with God.

So I ask that, when exploring this matter, you shift your attention towards your spirituality rating and not your religious rating. Not necessarily forever, just for the purpose of this program. Ideally, they would be they same rating.

A most comforting thought to me is that most religions believe the soul is eternal, which sounds good to me. Anyone in doubt of life after death should explore near death experiences.(I do not mean this literally!) The personal accounts of this phenomenon are the closest evidence we have to an after-life. Even if this phenomenon is somehow explained be a scientific anomaly, I still look forward to experiencing this "beyond blissful state," even if it is only for a moment. Fearing death and life after death is not health promoting. Fear in general is definitely not health promoting and does not bring you closer to spirituality. It is love and faith that lead to wellness, not fear.

Larry Dossey has many books that clearly describe the benefits of praying and how having faith contributes positively to your health. So if you want complete wellness, religion and spirituality need to be addressed.

Who Am I

I find this an appropriate time to share a little bit of my background, because it is important for many of you to know. "Why should I listen to this guy or that lady, what do they know," is a thought that people usually first have when meeting someone new. However, I suggest it is more important to listen to the message and not to concentrate on the messenger, which is often hard to do, I must admit. But I am a Stephen Covey student and I practice the message of seeking first to understand and only then do I seek to be understood(which, I think, is an old Chinese proverb), mainly because I already know what I know, but I do not know what you know.

To put it simply, I walk the talk. If the person you look to for health matters is overtly overweight, smokes, drink alcohol, is obviously over-worked, or seems super stressed every time you see him/her, is this really who you should be paying money to and taking advice from? Would you take your car to be fixed by a mechanic who drives a broken down rust bucket?

I can honestly say that I have never put a cigarette or any illegal drug into my system. I will admit, when I was in sixth grade, I tried chewing tobacco because of peer pressure from my baseball buddies. But after intense feelings of pain and sickness to my stomach, I never did that again. I have never been drunk in my life. The most I have ever consumed was two wine coolers in a few hours, which I could count the occasions on one hand. (Well, maybe two hands, but not three hands, that's impossible.) I have been involved in organized sports throughout school, and have been regularly lifting weights since I was eighteen years old. I radically changed my diet at age twenty-two, which does not involve eating most animal products. Years before that, I stopped eating fast foods.

I am a general, big picture kind of person, and do not prefer fine-minute details. Which explains why I like wellness, because it incorporates everything. I am proud to say I have only loved one woman, and I have a very wonderful child. I love the work I do. I sleep great 95% of the time. I have many leisure activities I love to participate in. I enjoy spending time with my extended family, and I am now on a spiritual path that I am relishing.

A pivotal point in my life was when I took a psychology class in high school, which stimulated my brain and created a new hunger to explore these wellness topics. While most of my friends were having fun partying or vacationing after high school, that summer I enrolled in an upper division philosophy night class at the community college. I did not know it at the time, but it was probably one of the most difficult subjects a student could tackle.(Looking back on that time, I realize my inner intelligence was clearly guiding me toward college, and I was right to listen.) I sat in the back of the class and rarely spoke. I did not understand too much, but I enjoyed myself nonetheless.

This was the same time I decided to move away from hopes of becoming a local union laborer. In my life I operate from the premise that everything happens for a reason and on purpose. Which is now evident because I failed the engineer entrance exam by half a point. The sheet metal union never called. My friend in the sprinkler fitter business told me the work was too hard and that I should stay in school and have fun. That same summer, I got a job as a plumber's assistant which resulted in only one week of working with grumpy men and unpleasant raw material. I am grateful for all of these experiences.

In the fall, I started taking classes full-time at the College of San Mateo, and decided that this was not a bad place to spend some time, until I figured out what I would do with my life. Plus it kept my dad off my back. He was always trying to find a way to kick me out of the house, not because he didn't like me, rather, it would make me a man and show me responsibility, etc.(That's because he left home at an early age and became successful.) Well thank you mom for talking some sense into the man and buying me some time.

My dad was the opposite of most parents. He actually wanted me to drop out of college and to quit fooling around, in order to get a full-time job. A notion he finally gave up on when I was actually handed my Bachelors degree. Maybe he was using reverse psychology, knowing teenagers do the opposite of what their parents want them to do. Although, my intuition tells me to very seriously doubt this was his intention. Don't get me wrong, I love my pops dearly and I hold absolutely no ill feelings toward him at all, I understand now where he was coming from.

While fooling around in community college, I stumbled onto Occupational Therapy. Although I did not know anyone who did this type of work, and only read briefly about it, this profession just fit with what I wanted to do with my life. What I wanted was to help others on a personal basis, in many aspects.

43

Occupational Therapists(O.T.'s) are trained in rehabilitation. Some examples would be providing rehabilitation services for premature infants, children with cerebral palsy, adults with work injuries, seniors with strokes, and all sorts of other physical and mental difficulties. My intention was not to become an O.T. forever. My main focus was to obtain diverse knowledge in the medical field. Classes ranged from kinesiology, neuroanatomy /physiology, various psychiatric and physical disability courses, and internships at hospitals. I loved them all.

It definitely was not an easy road, but I did receive my BS in O.T. from San Jose State University. I started this two-and-one-half-year program, while at the same time having my child at age twenty-three, working part-time, and living with Dori, the love of my life. Looking back, I only see this time as joyful.

All of these life events have led me toward wellness. Wellness is my bliss, my passion, it brings me happiness and peace. I study it and live it. Please let me conclude by stating that I am not "Super Wellness Man." There are surely many people on a higher wellness path than I. Again, the main point to remember is that we are on the right path-- moving in the right direction. Having said all of this, I hope you can put faith in the fact that you are indeed listening to someone who walks the wellness talk.

Finding Spirituality

In regard to my spirituality past, I went to "Our Lady of Mercy" Catholic grammar school for eight years. I do not regret going there at all. I loved the kids, parents, and teachers. However, I never bought into their religious teachings. I went along with it for a while, but slowly moved away from the church in that fifth grade when I chose not to become an altar boy. However, I did become an altar boy in the sixth grade, only because all my friends got to take a day off school to attend the altar boy picnic, while I stayed in class with all the girls.

In the eighth grade, I chose not to be confirmed. I would have been the only one to do so.(Except for one girl who was Asian, and only went to the school because it was private and not because of the religious aspect.) But I experienced a lot of arm twisting from my parents, so I reluctantly received confirmation.(Although, I do not remember what confirmation means.) I do not have any anger as a result of this experience because I learned from it.(Plus, the bishop rubbed some oil on my head.) I am grateful for this experience because it taught me the purpose of donating my time to help serve others in need. (Everything happens for a reason, and today I belong to a community service organization which I will later plug.)

I knew what was not benefiting me, and that was the teaching that Jesus Christ is the only way to God. I would always ask myself, "If Jesus Christ is the only way, then what about all those other people in the world who do not even know he existed, someone on a remote island, how could this guy get to heaven if he didn't pray to Jesus?"

Even as an adolescent I wondered, "What if I was born in India and not America, then I might have been a Hindu and worshipped cows." To me, religion was simply a matter of chance. If you are a devout Christian, you may be confidently thinking that I am *not yet ready* to allow Jesus into my life, and maybe you are correct, but up until now this has not been a consideration. I will stop here so I do not get myself into trouble.

The ideas of purgatory and hell did not seem beneficial to me, but I was hung up with the teachings that my soul would go there and not to heaven, if I wasn't a good boy. Maybe I just thought I was too mischievous to be a good boy, and I didn't want to work hard enough to get to heaven, so I gave up and convinced myself that the solution was not to believe in life after death.

After grammar school, I completely turned away from the church. All of my friends went to the large religious high schools, and I was the only one bold enough to know that although I would miss my friends dearly, this was not the path I wanted to be a part of.

(And at the time, these high schools didn't allow girls!)

If I was no longer a Catholic, then what was I ? I needed a new identity. That is when I learned about the concept of being an agnostic. I was a doubter of God's existence, but not an atheist. But as you know, I am a learner and I was not against finding out information about different religions. I was an agnostic for many years, until I went on vacation to Hawaii.

Going to Hawaii for the first time definitely changed my scope of spirituality. I learned the dichotomy of the Hawaiian practice of going to Christian churches regularly and yet believing in gods like Pele(the volcano goddess). It was very difficult, at first, not to see this as hypocritical. It was then that I slowly wondered if the way to move away from agnosticism was to move in the direction of animism. I new I had to move in the direction of something, because the more I learned in life, the more I knew that being a doubter was not benefiting me. The fact that the people in my life I considered to be my mentors--all believed in God, led me in a new direction also.

Self-Love

Whichever spiritual path you choose, self-love is a key to unlocking your full spiritual potential. There is a saying you may be familiar with, which is, "The eyes are windows to the soul." I would like to explore this phrase. Do you find it difficult to make eye contact with new people you meet and even those closest to you? Do you rub your eyes, yawn, look away frequently, or act like you are busy when others are trying to look into your soul? Doing so prevents your spirituality from connecting with others. A connection that we need. If this is a challenge for you, I suggest, as I learned from Louise Hay, that you get very close to a mirror and look directly into your iris and pupils and say the words "I love you." Say it as often as necessary until it feels like the absolute truth. You can use this same mirror to say anything positive to yourself. Give this a try, it cannot hurt. Perhaps doing this will allow you and others into the window of your soul. The soul that you are here on earth to discover and nourish. The soul that is one with the creator. Being able to do this mirror exercise is a good indication of your own self-love.

Another way to get closer to self-love would be to spend time with a pet or a five-month-old baby. These two beings do not judge you, and the only thing they see is your perfection. If you can give and receive unconditional love with them, then it will be easier to give and receive unconditional love with yourself.

How can someone claim to be close to God and to love God if they do not have complete self-love. To me, the two are one in the same. And once self-love is revealed, the sky is the limit.

Back on the Road

The question I would like to now pose to your intuition is:

"Are you on the road you have created, or are you on the road that your parents created, or the road your preacher created, or the road a holy book created?"

Maybe after a deep exploration of your spiritual beliefs, you may come to the pleasing conclusion that you are indeed part of the right religious group, *for you*, after all. Or you may come to the alarming realization that you want to move in a new direction.

If your current spiritual beliefs are not serving you, then change them. Why would someone practice a spiritual life in which they are in constant unhappiness. To me this makes no sense. You are not bound by any belief you have had in the past. If you do not know how to create a working spiritual model in your life, that is OK. There are many people who have written on this subject, for thousands of years, all over the world! There is bound to be one that fits *your* true beliefs. If not, then start your own group of similar thinking spiritual mindbodies. (Maybe I should not have said that, I don't want to be responsible for another Hale-Bop incident.)

I believe that everything I have done in life has been perfect and has been leading up to this point, this writing, this message. Having said that, I have to admit I heard the very passionate and witty Mariann Williamson say something toady that really hit a chord with me. She insisted we are all here to first discover our message, and then we are to share this message with others. And this is a vital reason I am, and we all are, here on earth. The striking blow to my bodymind set is that she thinks it is not so important to share this message with millions of people or the whole world(which is what my multi-lingual ego wants), but that it is equally and perhaps even more important to share this message with those that are in my life right now. My innate intelligence tells me she is correct. Thank you Mariann.

Forcing your religion on another person is no more appropriate than forcing any wellness belief on another. All you can do is share the message with another. I am going to allow my daughter the unique opportunity of discovering her own spiritual path. Certainly I will guide her with human values and principled ethics, but if I take her to one church, I better take her every church or temple in town. I have enough confidence in her to know that she too will find her message in life, and she will share it with others. But I do not have to find her message for her. I simply need to provide the opportunity for her to discover the message.

I am now back on the road. The road of the spirituality that I was born with. I do not have a name or label for my specific beliefs, I just have feelings. This is why I choose to use the word spirituality instead of religion. And in the end, it would seem more beneficial for everyone to at least work off the same basic feelings, which is that *all roads lead to God*, even the road of the atheist. Of all wellness areas, I would tend to think there is only one way to find and maintain a rating of ten, and that would be to reach the big house in the sky, because spirituality is a never ending exploration.

Let me end this chapter by throwing out two final questions to ponder.

1. "How can you *really* know God until you have not known God?"

> If you have always known God, then you are lucky indeed. I took the long road.

2."Why is spirituality so important for achieving wellness?"

Just ask someone who had no spiritual direction or beliefs for a very long time, and now they do, now they have found their path.

The importance is evident, you can see it in their eyes and feel it in their presence!

CHAPTER 5
LEISURE

I do know a little something about this wellness topic, as I worked for my local park and recreation department throughout high school and college. I even considered a career in this field, except the pay was too low and the job market was unstable. I performed numerous job duties including recreation leader, officiating athletic leagues, facilitating party rentals, and participating in various community events. I also put together a few adult softball teams. This is not meant to be a resume. It is meant to show that I have seen the benefits that recreation and leisure have created for children and adults, boys and girls. I witnessed the transformation people would go through, it is almost indescribable. Kids and adults that were very shy and timid were allowed the opportunity to freely express their spirit with themselves and others.

We need leisure, strictly fun time, in our lives. Hopefully every wellness area is more fun than not. However, leisure should always be fun 100% of the time. Leisure can be whatever you want it to be. I really don't think I need to list one hundred different ways to experience leisure. Leisure can be anything, but it better be something. Leisure activities can give you true insight to yourself. The fun and loving you. The care free, time is flying by--you.

There are two kinds of leisure, passive and active. Do you have a balance between the two? Passive leisure would be things like watching television and listening to music. These examples do not usually require active participation and they do not provide a challenge. You may consider going to the coffee shop to read the newspaper as active leisure, but I see this as passive. Technically you could argue that going to the mall is active, but it does not require much involvement or thinking.

Passive leisure is not a bad thing. We need time in our lives when we can kick-back and simply relax, but we do not need it in excess. Active leisure activities will bring more happiness as it requires your focused attention and it provides feedback. Some examples would be sports, art projects, and preparing a new dinner recipe.

I propose that we need to balance both active and passive leisure to expand wellness. It is certainly possible to have too much emphasis on any wellness area, including leisure. There is a small culture of surfers that literally live hand-to-mouth, going around the world to ride the big waves, for years on end. My guess is if anyone was ever to do a wellness study on this group of free spirits, we would eventually see a trend of compromised health.

I hope by now we have all experienced the joys of leisure. These experiences create lasting emotions, and it is emotions that we remember and carry around with us. If you spend all your time worrying and feeling pressured, then these are the emotions you will remember and carry around with you. As an adult, hopefully you can look back on the fun childhood adventures of going on vacations, to amusement parks, camping, or going on picnics. Unfortunately, I realize that some kids were not provided these leisure opportunities and experiences. However, we cannot change the past, and now is the time to create those experiences to imbed new positive emotions into your bodymind so you can start to carry these around with you instead.

Make time for leisure, put it in your appointment book, write it in your calendar, don't get around to it later. How much time should you schedule? Everyday would be nice! If reading novels is your favorite all-time leisure activity, then do it everyday, even if it is one chapter or even one page. Only you know how much time you need to feel good and satisfied in this area. And you also know that making no time at all is probably not what your intuition is asking for.

How about doing something you have always wanted to try, but for some reason you make excuses to avoid it. If you always wondered what it would be like to surf, then go to the beach and talk to some surfers. If you have been curious about what it would be like to hit a golf ball, borrow a friend's clubs and start hacking away. If you are drawn toward learning how to make ceramic sculptures, go sign up for a class at the local community college. Your success is not based on how good the end result is, success is the actual joy producing process. All of these steps are simple, inexpensive, and fun. Whatever you do, do something.

Vacation

One question I ask my patients, friends, and most acquaintances is, "When was the last time you went on vacation, and when is your next one planned." Sometimes I get a laugh or a huge sigh. If they cannot easily remember the last vacation they took, or if they say they haven't had one for years, with no future plans for a vacation, I consider this to be something in need of immediate attention.

I have a patient, we will call her Emma, that I am treating for a spinal fusion of her lumbar vertebrae, as a result of three ruptured discs. She has a long history of back pain, Parkinson's, and rheumatoid arthritis. When I asked her about anything related to wellness, such as leisure time and vacations, all of her answers were directly related to the fact that she did not have time for most wellness areas, because she was always taking care of an ill family member. She has literally been taking care of everyone from her brother with Hodgkin's disease, to her long lost cousin that had a stroke, for the last thirty-five years. Although she seems very nice and attractive, she never made time for marriage and never had children.

I am currently reading *Awakening Intuition*, by Dr. Mona Lisa Schultz. Amazingly, she explains how all of the problems

51

Emma has, are directly related to her emotional need to be in control, which is correlated to "The first emotional center" called "Blood and Bones." Emma suffers from "The Eggs-In-One Basket Syndrome." All of her life revolves around taking care of her family members. These family members gave away their control to Emma and she took it. I believe all of Emma's illnesses are definitely influenced by her emotional complexities. It is certainly noble that she has been a trusted relative, but she has never had a break long enough to make time for herself and to experience pure leisure or a real vacation.

Vacations do not have to be extravagant or cost big bucks. A vacation can be whatever you want it to be. I live in the San Francisco Bay Area, and many people often take a quick getaway to Lake Tahoe or Reno, to gamble. But I find that for some reason they tend not to consider this to be a real vacation.(Regardless of whether they won money or not.) By simply shifting your focus from making this a waste of time and money, you can choose to see it as only fun, like the beautiful drive, the fancy hotel lights, the nice people, and the endless buffets. To me, this is a vacation. Whether it was one day or seven, I still made time for leisure and felt fabulous about it.

This year I have scheduled three camping trips throughout California, and I invited all my family and friends.(Knowing that some would not find leisure as a priority, hopefully someone will attend.) The cost is minimal and the fun is endless. For me, leisure is such a regular and natural part of my being, it is hard to imagine anyone who would feel different. Maybe they feel they do not deserve it or must spend more time sacrificing for their kids, work, and everything and everyone else first. In case no one ever gave you permission before, I will take the liberty of now giving you permission. Be selfish for one hour, for one day, with no guilt.

If you always go to the same vacation spot every year, how about trying a new place this year. Pull out the globe or a map, this will help you to see the big picture. Leisure is another fairly safe way to be spontaneous, so spin the globe or the map, close your eyes, and wherever your finger is pointed when it stops, is *your* next stop. And if no one wants to go where you want to, go by yourself. I have an uncle who takes vacations all over the world by himself. He only has to focus on his own experience and fun, and always has a marvelous time.

I do not think I need to write tons of examples of why and how leisure is related to wellness, do you? All of our ancestors participated in leisure activities and so should you. Trial and error, and your intuition will lead the way.

One way to bring more wellness to your life is to combine leisure with fitness. And really, shouldn't your main fitness outlet be considered leisurable also? Think about this as we head into the fitness arena.

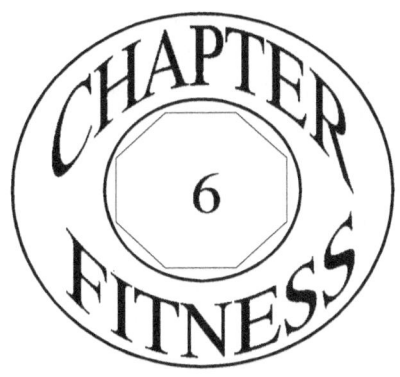

CHAPTER 6 FITNESS

I suspect by now that we are all used to hearing every health related expert, book, and magazine tell us how and why we need to exercise. There are enormous amounts of studies in the medical literature linking the benefits of proper and regular exercise to all of the wellness areas mentioned in this book. My intuition frankly tells me that these studies are correct. How about your intuition?

One example of the benefits of participating in a fitness program is the relationship between depression and exercise. When I did my internship at the Menninger acute psychiatric ward, I led a morning exercise session for the patients. At first, I was skeptical of the purpose for doing this group. However, it was truly amazing to see how these depressed people(who on the outside--look like you and I) would start to smile more, make more eye contact, and begin to talk about their problems. All of this, simply by standing in a circle and doing a few stretches. I am not suggesting this exercise group cured them, but it was definitely a major component of returning them to a more balanced state.

I personally know a woman, we will call her Julia, who is forty-seven years old, and has been very depressed with various mind/body illnesses for many years. She has been sulking over a divorce that happened five years ago, she was obviously over-weight, could not keep a job, has a problem child, and the list literally goes on and on. Six months ago she took a job at a fitness center, as a janitor. I recently saw her for the first time in over one year. I was flabbergasted to say the least.

Julia is now at a normal weight. I can finally see what it looks like to have a smile come from her face. She does not sleep on the couch all day long, anymore. Her eating habits have tremendously improved, and she is now going to church regularly.

Can you guess what happened to cause such dramatic changes to occur? Julia not only began to work at the gym, she was talked into lifting weights with one of the personal trainers. She has now worked out many of her problems in life by "working-out." She is actually considering entering in an amateur body building contest, next year. Last year, I would have bet a days pay against seeing her participate in any fitness program whatsoever. All of her problems were not cured, but believe me, I am not exaggerating when I say she is a new woman, now that she exercises regularly.

Finding Fitness

Throughout evolution, we were always provided plenty of opportunity to exercise, except back then it was in the form of work, war, migrating, gathering, hunting, and farming. Only until this century have we moved away from an active lifestyle, mainly as a result of modern technology. We do not need to walk miles every day to find food anymore. All we have to do is walk up and down a few shopping isles, then drive home in the car and sit for several hours at a desk or on the telephone.

Fancy equipment and high cost is not a pre-requisite for fulfilling your fitness area. If you like going to a fitness center and using high-tech machines, then continue to do so. The simplest, cheapest, and most natural form of obtaining adequate exercise is walking.

Everyone knows how to do this, you do not need a trainer, and there is a very low risk for injury. You can do it most anywhere and anytime, with anyone. You can go at any pace you wish to stride for. You can walk the dog, or if you don't have one, then walk the neighbors dog. You can listen to the radio. You can walk up a hill or on the beach. And you can simply enjoy the beauty nature has provided.

Experts in the fitness field have come up with very specific advice on how to measure your exact fitness level. These measurements are easy to find in any fitness guide. However, I think our intuition can also let us know what a healthy fitness level should be. My inner self tells me, when I play basketball after a three month hiatus, that when I start to suck air so badly that my chest hurts and my legs feel like rubber, after only ten minutes, I am not at my usual fitness level. I know this because I did not usually feel these bodily discomforts until after playing for forty-five minutes.

A general rule of thumb is that if your heart feels like it is jumping out of your chest and you cannot even say 911, then you are working too hard. Ideally you should at least break a slight sweat and your breathing rate should increase so you can still carry on a short conversation. Although sitting on the beach, in the sauna or in the steam room are great ways to release toxins and stress, and will produce perspiration, don't think you are tricking your rishi into thinking you are exercising. You cannot fool the knower inside.

Do I Have to Exercise?

Making enough time for regular exercise may not be physically necessary for some people. For example, a mail carrier walks several miles each day, sometimes up and down large hills, as a part of their duties. A park ranger who gives generous hiking tours may travel several miles daily. Most UPS workers are extremely fit. In fact, I knew a guy who worked at 3 AM busting his tail off at UPS, and then later that same day, I would regularly see him doing high impact aerobics at the gym!

When I lived in Hilo-Hawaii, we rented a nice home with a good sized yard, full of overgrown greenery, left from the renter before us. On my days off, I would go outside with the clippers, saw, and garbage bags. I would sometimes find myself lost in such a state that my wife would beg me to come inside already and take a break. I was a city boy and never had to do any gardening work before, so I thought cleaning the yard would be quick and easy. However, I was exhausted and full of sweat with fatigued muscles and a strong pumping heart, in less than one hour. I not only gained a new appreciation for the fitness level required for such work, but I also developed a new leisure activity because I loved creating a masterpiece with a few tools and some imagination.

Anything physical can be considered a fitness activity if it makes you sweat and increases your heart rate. Actually, an active monogamous sex life could even be considered a good form of toning your fitness, assuming you perform more than a one minute warm up and less than an eight hour cool down.

Too Tired to Exercise

Some of you might find it easier to avoid exercising by telling yourself, because you are on your feet all day long, you do not need to workout. If you are a school teacher you may be on your feet all day and feel tired at the end of the day. But you were probably never short of breath(except for talking too much), your heart rate never significantly increased(except for when little Jimmy pulled the fire alarm), and your flexibility may not have been challenged(except when pulling apart two wrestling kids.) Being on your feet most of the day probably did not do much for your strength and endurance.(Maybe initially it did, if you were used to sitting down all day in class yourself, and studying to become a teacher for years before.)

Improving your energy level for fitness will automatically improve when the other seven wellness levels are improved, because all areas support each other. Your energy resources are like your money resources. You have to put money into the bank, in order to draw it out when you need to spend it. The more you put in, the more you can take out. But if you put your money in a passbook savings account, you will not make as much as you would from putting it in a money market account. If you put your energy into things like worrying needlessly and stressing over things you have no control over, you will have less energy needed for more important ventures and adventures.

Feeling too tired to exercise and not making the time are probably the two major reasons some people do not fulfill this wellness requirement. I find, and have heard from many others, that once you actually get started in the activity, then the rest of the workout becomes much easier. Just knowing this fact helps me when I search for excuses to put exercise off. I might say to myself, "Come on Jim, put down the book and pick up the barbell, after your first set you won't want to put it down."

On the other side of the coin, I remember when I first started lifting weights, I went overboard from the "lifters high." One day I walked in the gym, sat down on the bench, put my hands on the barbell, looked at it and let out a huge sigh, got up and went home. I was burnt out. I was going to the gym five times a week for a full year without a break. I did not return for one month and began to pay more attention to my instinct.

Increasing your fitness level can only add to your wellness strength. The only caveat would be the potential for injury as a result of ignoring your senses. If the fitness program you participate in is causing sharp pains, you should stop doing whatever it is that is causing the pain, even if that means letting this activity go and starting a new one. Please don't work through the sharp pain until it goes away. You can have gain without pain. Ignoring adequate warm up and cool down, not practicing proper technique, and overuse are usually related to the pain, not the exercise itself.

Personally, I have been regularly lifting weights for nine years. I like to: walk with my family and my dog, ride my bicycle around town, play golf(I walk the course, I do not take a cart), perform various stretches, play basketball periodically, and I boogie board when I go to Hawaii. This last sport requires a very good fitness level, so be careful!(By the way, please do not ever try boogie boarding without a wet suit in the San Francisco Bay, unless you want to know what you would look like as a purple Popsicle. Believe me, it was not fun.)

Posture

I was labeled a slouch throughout school because of my posture. You know, the typical rounded shoulders and kyphotic posture of the Hunchback of Notre Dame. One of the main purposes I started to lift weights was to specifically address my poor posture. Weight-lifting really did make noticeable improvements, even to this day.

Recently I read books on the topic of "Feldenkrais" and "The Alexander Technique." Both therapies teach proper movement and facilitate balanced posture. I have been integrating these principles the past few months and have gained wonderful benefits from them. For instance, now I refrain from leaning against the back of any chair, and I cue myself to walk with my head up, instead of looking at the ground. Especially when walking down the street, I remind myself to smile and make eye contact with the person walking toward me, as opposed to looking away. I now allow my buttocks and my femurs to hold me upright when sitting in a chair, as opposed to sitting on my tailbone.

If one part of your body is not aligned, this will have the tendency to throw the rest of your body out of alignment. Your head position is key. If you are always looking at the floor when walking, then your spine flexes, which makes your pelvis shift, which leads your knees to be out of position, and your feet may turn inward or outward to provide more stability for this awkward walking style. All of this, just because you were looking down. Developing and maintaining good posture is wellness promoting. Your organs and joints will not be crushed and your body will be more toned and balanced. It will also do wonders for your self-confidence.

Unless you have been living under a rock, I am sure you understand the necessity for having a strong fitness level. Please see the chapters about time and change to get you motivated to integrate this wellness area into your lifestyle forever. One way to be more motivated for fitness is to have fun exercising with family and friends. Let us now look at how to bring balance to this wellness area.

CHAPTER 7

FAMILY & FRIENDS

A lthough this chapter appears in the middle of the book, I actually wrote about this topic last. Why? Perhaps I was waiting for my intuition to jumpstart me. The other reason may be that this subject can be such an individual, complicated, and emotional matter to describe, I wanted to be highly focused before I attempted to make any sense of it.

"What do my family and friends have to do with my wellness?"

As you know, human beings are social beings. No person is an island. We need each other to survive. We need each other to create and maintain wellness. It is that simple. Newborn babies void of touch, will become very sick physically and mentally, as opposed to babies who are given plenty of hugs and kisses. The same reality is true for adults who are deficient of close relationships.

One reason we have forgotten about how much we need the closeness of others is that we are living in an individualistic and technologic society. We are taught that we need to move away from home right after school to take on the world, alone in an apartment, as opposed to living in a multi-generational household. We are supposed to have our own vehicle, instead of using public transportation or carpooling. (To me it makes more sense to stay close to home, and to contribute my resources to the town I live in, instead of somebody else's town!) We use drive-through fast food windows so we can eat in our cars alone, therefore we do not have to eat with others, which is totally opposite of our cultural evolution.

We all have some form of family and friends available to us. Even someone who has no living relatives and just moved to a new town, has the option of creating a new set of friends and family. The terms family and friends can actually mean the same thing. For instance, many people consider their spouse to be their best friend, myself included. In Hawaii, people call everybody who is close to them grandma, auntie, uncle, or brother, whether they are blood relatives or not. The amazing thing is that the people use these words as if they were literal, not just figuratively. And they may not care to spend any time with actual blood relatives at all. They just know they like to be around and feel close to certain people, the rest is a technicality.

Love

Several years ago I stumbled onto the teachings of a man I call the love doctor, Leo Buscalia, a passionate and famous Italian that speaks about love and families. He sparked my awareness to find a way to bring my family closer together. For some of you the concept of a "family meeting" is normal. But my family never did this, and I felt it would be a nice way to initiate open communication. We have been holding this meeting once a year, after Thanksgiving dinner. I think these meetings are perfect, and they have evolved from yelling matches, into a peaceful-loving support group. (Well, not quite that extreme.) Although everybody sort of sarcastically says, "Oh no, not the family meeting again," my inner intelligence tells me they too enjoy it. Maybe you would like to start a family tradition to bring your family closer together. Give it a try, there has got to be something that works.

Something that has worked for me was an idea I got from a friend at work. At the beginning of this year I asked my wife, "Hunny, do you want to make a New Year's resolution with me?" She immediately rolled her eyes and let out a huge sigh while stating, "Oh boy, not one of your wellness things again." Much to her surprise, I proposed that we start a new tradition of going out on a date, alone-without the baby, once a month. This was a challenging goal, as we had probably averaged one date a year since Noelani was born. The first month went by and we didn't go on the date. Although we had talked about it, we neglected to set aside the time. But as you know, in the wellness scheme of things, you never fail until you stop trying, and the important message is that you are moving in the right direction. So the next month we agreed to actually schedule the date and make babysitting plans at the beginning of the month. At the time of this writing we have made six dates in a row, and it is becoming a regular habit for us to spend quality time together. A habit that I intend on keeping forever.

Love can be a complicated subject at times, as many great thinkers have attempted to define it and explain it for thousands of years. I suppose we all have different ideas about what love is. Some people sit around and complain that nobody loves them therefore they cannot give love to anyone else. I believe we all have love inside of us, it is natural. As I already eluded to, true love first comes from self-love. If you have true self-love, then you can give love to others. I simply operate from the knowing that what goes around comes around. I give love freely, without conditions, and I can see love coming back to me throughout the day.

For instance, I tell my daughter I love her, literally a dozen times a day, because that is how I truly feel. But I never ask her if she loves me. I don't tell her I love her eagerly waiting for her to say I love you back. And it may not surprise you to know that this four year old beauty comes up to me at various times and gives me a big hug and voluntarily tells me she loves me.

Love is body and mind. Saying I love you is important and so is showing it physically. I have never had someone deny me a hug when I asked for it. I remember being at a huge outdoor concert at Golden Gate Park and there was a young man with a sign written on his body that read "Free Hugs." I watched this guy for one hour as he repeatedly shouted "Free Hugs" and over one hundred people, men and women, gave him a big hug. I liked his idea and ever since that day, I use the phrase "Free Hugs" when I feel someone needs some love, and when I feel I need some love.

You Make the Call

Not all relationships are ideal, and sometimes we wish we could undo the past. If you are contemplating making amends with the past in order to become closer to your friends and family, there is a good chance they too would like to wipe the slate clean. Besides, if you are not at peace with the past, that means you are spending less time focusing on today. You must be bold enough to be the first one to reach out. If the other person does not reach back, that is OK too. It is not beneficial to feel rejected or to take it personal. The truth is that the other person was simply *not ready*, but at least they know where you stand, and the ball is now in their court. I have a very vivid example that depicts a situation of reaching out.

My wife Dori never knew her father. He never took responsibility for his child, and even if he intended on doing so someday, he died when she was eight years old. She literally never knew anything about this side of her family, and her mother was not forthcoming in the matter. This was until she graduated high school, when one of her dad's sisters tried to contact Dori. She chose not to talk to the aunt, and was not sure why after all these years, she now wanted to make contact.

Every year or so, I would hint around to Dori about the possibility of contacting her dad's family, but Dori would not want to discuss this, and she would get upset when I would broach the subject. To me this was frustrating. I was more willing to find out about her family than she was. The thought of having a brother or sister and not knowing them, seemed outrageous to me. But over time, I began to understand the pain she associated from having a father who never did his job. Dori did not have a very close relationship with her mother either. Combine this with the fact that Dori was here in California while most all of her mother's side of the family was in Hawaii, was an obvious gap in her family wellness area, contributing to poor balance in her overall health.

Again this year, I brought up the topic, and she surprisingly asked for my help into finding her long lost *ohana*.(This means family in Hawaiian.) I actually had to hire a private investigator to find her dad's widow. The investigator only came up with an address that was three years old. Dori mailed her a nice letter, basically saying that she wanted to establish a relationship and was eager to learn about her father, not knowing if her father's widow would even get this letter.

A week or so later, Dori anxiously went to the mailbox one night, somehow knowing there would be a response to her letter. The family was ecstatic to receive Dori's letter, and they swear that they had planned to find Dori that same week.

It turns out Dori has two younger sisters and an older brother. And her dad and his wife and kids actually lived here in Stockton right before he died. Also, Dori and her sisters went to the same schools in Hawaii, but at different times. Even more uncanny is that her dad's brother lives only twenty minutes away, two aunts live ninety minutes away from us, and the auntie that tried to contact Dori after graduation, lives in Southern California. On top of all this, the next week we were invited to a "get together" that was already scheduled, where we got to meet all of her aunts, uncle, and some cousins. They are all very wonderful people, and they helped us to learn about the family.

If this whole scenario isn't synchronicity, then I don't know what is! As a result, Dori has filled the gap that prevented peace in her life, and she now has a sparkle in her eyes that could light up the night sky. The point of this story is to show how you never know when you'll find an uncle in your own backyard. Actually, it is to show how it is very difficult to have wellness forever--without everyone.

Don't wait until you are on your death bed to make peace with your family and friends in order to ease your conscience. Make amends today. Tell your family and friends that you love them and that you feel lucky to have them in your life, assuming you *truly* feel this way.(Always tell the truth, because truth is wellness, lying is dis-ease.)

Look them in the eye and say this as you give love freely without expectations of getting love back.

Communication

We need family and friends to give and receive wellness support. One way we show support is by open communication. This means active listening, and understanding that speaking or giving advice comes secondary, even if your ego wants its view to be the primary reason for engaging in conversation. You can give advice, but it is usually more effective when it is asked for first. Giving unsolicited advice will usually not prove to be immediately effective. Instead, after listening attentively to your friend, although your ego wants to jump up and tell your friend what to do, you might subtly say something like, "I too have encountered the same sort of situation," or "I used to think that way before, also." This opens the door for advice, as we all want to help our loved ones. But you must also remain aware of how the human ego wants to think it figured things out on its own.

This is evident when it comes to parenting. Do not ever give a parent unsolicited advice about how to raise their children, unless you are looking for enemies. Personally, I like to ask people about different parenting ideas, not only because I am a rookie at this job, but also because I know parents like to brag about their child's good habits. Everyone loves to be asked for advice, don't you? You do not have to feel like you are sounding ignorant by asking questions, especially to strangers. Asking for someone's opinion, opens the door to communication.

The truth is that learning about relationships and increasing open communication is just as important as learning about nutrition or any other wellness area. Unfortunately, your ego may prevent you from listening to something like *Men are from Mars and Women are from Venus,* by John Gray. "I do not need to listen to some monk tell me how to love my wife," yells Mr. Tough Guy. Well, John Gray must be saying something reasonable because millions of people have benefited from his views, including me. That does not mean you should follow everything a famous author teaches. These experts simply provide tools, and if the tools work, then use them, if not, then throw them away.

When communicating, disagreements are bound to arise. Friendly arguments can be fun when new dilemmas arise, but having the same bitter arguments every day for thirty years is not fun. Why do we sacrifice time, energy, and love to have meaningless arguments when we could be using that time for hugging, kissing, playing, and sharing? Whether the bed got made, car got washed, or toilet seat was left up doesn't matter, they are all meaningless. If the person wanted to do these tasks then they would have done them. In Hawaii the locals operate on "Hawaiian time," which means if something doesn't get done today as planned, "no matter," just do it tomorrow. Sometimes tomorrow could mean weeks or months.

I love to have spirited debates, but lately I have moved away from meaningless arguments, like whether or not my daughter has on matching socks. If she wanted to match her socks, she *would* match her socks. So why does it upset my wife so much when Noe chooses to wear one blue and one yellow sock? To me this is a waste of time. She could make the same argument every day for ten years and the odds that I would change my outlook would be next to nil. Think about this the next time you insist on changing someone else's meaningless point of view.

Making the Time

The third key component to the friends and family wellness area, including love and communication, is time. It is difficult to exchange love and to communicate with others if you do not make the time to do so. I am referring to quality time, of course. You can spend years in a house together with a sibling or spouse and never achieve a close relationship. You can always choose your friends but you cannot always choose your family members. The same rule applies that all you can do is offer to make the quality time, but you cannot force them to take you up on the offer. I already gave several examples of how I have chosen to set aside specific time for my loved ones, and there are more examples in chapter eleven.

On the other hand, some friends and family members are definitely not conducive to wellness, like abusers and criminals. You need to give them your love and tell them that you will help when they are ready. Sometimes the hardest thing to do is to step away from the relationship. You need to refrain from self-blame and the thinking: "If I only tried harder then they would have come around and seen the light."

You first and foremost have to be aware of your own wellness, and how staying in a dangerous relationship is breaking down your health. Remaining in these relationships will only produce two people with poor health, instead of one. You can't help someone who is not ready. **When the student is ready, the teacher will appear**, I guarantee it!

The topic of family and friends segues nicely into the wellness career area, as many of our close relationships revolve around work, and it is with your family that you share the happenings at work. And some families have businesses together, including me.

CHAPTER 8 CAREER

When I walk into a new patient's room, I smile and introduce myself as Jim Dennis the Occupational Therapist. "Your doctor wants me to help you," I say in an endearing manner. I often get a response of, " Thank you son, but I don't need a job anymore, I am retired."

The dictionary's definition of *occupation* is; an activity in which a person is engaged. Essentially, occupation can also be described as everything you ever do in life, which is what the wellness model I am presenting is all about, your whole life.

Occupational Therapy philosophies are based on the observations that we are all built to perform meaningful and purposeful activities/functions. And when people get sick, they stop engaging in these functions, which are also known as activities of daily living or ADL's. It can often be hard to find meaning and purpose in life when you are lying flat on your back in a compromised condition. So the basic premise is that if I can get the patient out of bed or off the couch, or at the very least to perform simple activities in bed, they will once again have the opportunity to perform life activities which will help to facilitate recovery.

I am not talking about doing exercises one-two-three, these are not necessarily ADL's. Getting dressed, taking a shower, feeding yourself, and writing your name are some common examples of basic ADL's. Higher level ADL's would be things like working or driving a car.

I know this all sounds like a plug for my profession, however, the main point is that we are all built to work, to have a career. The dictionary states that *career* is: an occupation followed as one's lifework. In the early history of humans, a caveperson's lifework was gathering and hunting to survive. Over time we evolved lifework to not only survive, but to barter goods. And today our lifework is still to trade goods, but with the exchanging of monies with each other, with less emphasis on survival. My point is that the money came last. Which to me means that money is not the priority for one's lifework. For modern day society, a career can literally be anything you can think of. School can also be considered a career for kids and even for adults.

Flowing to Bliss

Whatever you do for a living can be wonderful, as long as you feel you are being productive. And what you do must have meaning and some purpose you can see. In his book *Flow,* Mihaly Csikszentmihalyi discovers how some people can perform work in such a state, that there is no concept of time. The person is deeply engulfed in the task, and they are absolutely experiencing pure bliss. This can be true for any wellness area, not just your career. A great night's sleep is like experiencing "flow." You fall asleep at 10 PM and wake up at 7 AM, but you were not waking up every five minutes asking yourself if it was 7 AM yet, you simply enjoyed the act of sleeping.

I think one difficulty some people have with their career is that they have a job in which they do not have "flow" experiences. And just when they find that "flow" experience, they get the boot or the company down-sizes. Why? Because of modern day technology, one never knows when a machine is going to become the new employee.

Your career should be something you love to do, something you look forward to. I am not talking about becoming a workaholic. You are a workaholic if; you work extremely long hours, you need work as your main source of feeling good about yourself, you have high stress, and you do not allow time for other wellness activities. Being a workaholic is not part of a wellness lifestyle.

If you are one of these people with a new job every few months, it may not be because you are a bad worker, it may be that you are searching for that perfect "flow" career. There is something out there for you, I guarantee it! The awesome thing about our society is that we are not limited to working for someone else. You can create your own business. Millions have already done it, and you can too.

I deeply believe your intuition will help you discover your bliss and to pursue it. You can find your bliss career through trial and error, but this could take years. How about giving your "gut feeling" some respect, and cut to the chase. Your bliss career is something you would do for free for~every~one. And the word *vocation* means an activity to which one is called for reasons that go beyond earning a living. I somehow have always known that my bliss vocation is wellness. I share it with anyone, at anytime and any place. Are you sure of your bliss vocation?

Sometimes people know what their bliss career is, but they feel limited by a lack of knowledge or funds. If it was truly your bliss, there would not be any excuse that could stop you. Let's say you believe your bliss career is to be a politician.(God bless your soul.) If this was truly the case, there is no doubt that you could do it. Being a politician is truly your bliss only if the process is just as blissful as the end product. That means you will have to enjoy raising funds, public speaking, and reading literature about laws and regulations. The end goal may not be reached overnight, but if the entire process is blissful, you will never be disappointed.

Remember the movie *Field of Dreams*, and how the main character kept hearing a voice that was telling him to build a baseball field in the middle of his corn field? This seemed like the most bizarre thing he could do at the time. His family was struggling along on the farm, and he goes out on a limb and decides to follow his intuition. "Build it and he will come," is what the little voice inside his head was suggesting. Well, he built the baseball field, and his dad and the people came. Maybe they didn't come the second he finished it, but they did come. This is the kind of faith that you need to have when starting your own bliss career.

Once again, your bliss career can be anything. Although my neighbor Gloria is a grandmother, she is starting her own business after all these years. She is preparing an ice cream truck service. I wish you could see the enthusiasm she has in regard to all aspects of her career in the making. For example, she came over to our house and we helped her to design a flyer for "The Ice Cream Arena." It took my wife less than fifteen minutes to create the flyer, and I am not exaggerating when I say that I thought Gloria was going to explode with joy from holding this colorful piece of paper in her hands.

Her bliss is not merely driving around a big purple and white truck, her bliss is being able to bring joy to the children of the community. She enjoys the entire process. Whether your choice is to be a politician or an ice cream truck driver, both are equal because they are blissful.

A fun and easy book to help you get your own business started, without being overwhelmed, is called *Start Your Own Business in Thirty Days*, by Joseph Grappo.

You can also find numerous books on starting your own business, at the local library. You have to start somewhere. A reasonable goal is to slowly put together a business plan a few hours a week, while keeping your current mediocre job. It may take several months or a year but at least it should be fun(see chapter ten on goal setting.)

Haven't you heard the saying that you should follow your bliss. I take the phrase to heart. If you are working each day counting the hours and wondering how much money you made the last ten minutes, and could care less if the person you work for went belly up tomorrow, guess what!, you are in the wrong place. If your premise of life is happiness, you would have never reached this state in the first place.

For instance, writing this entire book was pure happiness, pure "flow." I never worried about what time it was or when it would end. Even if you are earning a million dollars a year from a career you find little pleasure in, you are cheating yourself if you do not follow your bliss. Wellness is bliss, wellness is not necessarily money. Following your bliss can only be a positive experience, even when it is *the road less traveled.*

Thinking you can separate your unhappiness at your job from the other wellness areas of your life is not realistic. How could someone go to a place every day and feel miserable, then expect to come home from work and pull a 180 and be Mr./Mrs. Entertainment to their children or spouse. This is not realistic. Being happy in your career should only lead to further happiness at home.

Volunteering

We are all made up of the same stuff of life. The same subatomic particles, the same body organs and functions. The same in 99% of all components of matter. Then why do some beings in this world focus negatively on the 1% difference?

Volunteering is a way to see the other 99% of the person, the 99% that is the same as you are, inside and out. It is a way to make a connection with the world in a unique fashion. Volunteering in the form of donating money is praise worthy, but that is not what I am suggesting here.

I had a recent "Aha" moment that I think fits well with this topic. A few years ago I heard Deepak Chopra speak on the science behind how a hologram is created, and I remember thinking at the time, "OK Deepak, so now I know how a hologram works, so what's the point?" What he was saying, but what I was *not ready* to comprehend, was the idea that everyone on earth is like a hologram. We are all whole beings and yet we are whole parts of a greater whole, which is our connection to each other and with God. So if you want to know God and the God inside you, then volunteering your services can only bring you closer to this knowing.

Human beings are built to do work, we were not necessarily built to work for money. Volunteering your time is a form of work, and seems admirable, but who has the time anymore(please see chapter eleven on time.) You can volunteer almost anywhere, at any time, doing any service you desire. (Sounds like a dream job--doesn't it?) Volunteering your time is actually selfish in a way. Most people report enjoying themselves and feeling good inside, when volunteering. Maybe even more-so than the people on the receiving end. Volunteering your services can only bring good karma.

I began to volunteer last year. I belong to an organization called SERTOMA which is an acronym for service to mankind. This group is community based. Our group decides on ways to raise money and then we vote on ways to appropriately distribute the funds to local charitable causes. I feel lucky to have found SERTOMA. As you might have guessed, because I love old folks, I am the youngest member by twenty years. Where are all of my peers? You do not have to be old and retired to belong to a civic service organization, or to give back to your community. I actually bring my four-year-old to many of the fundraisers and meetings. Believe it or not, she enthusiastically asks me, "When are we going to SERTOMA daddy?"

If you are undecided about joining a club like this, stop by a local SERTOMA meeting, they are all over North America. Or, be a trend setter and start a club in your hometown.

Another way my family volunteered was that we just finished hosting an Austrian student, who studied at The University of Pacific with thirty other kids from Austria and Germany. We had never done this before but we are very glad we did. The only difficult part of this experience was saying goodbye.

Again, volunteering in this fashion was as selfish, as it was giving. For me, communicating with someone from across the world is a thrill in itself, while on the internet. But to have this wonderful teenager share her worldly experiences with us was fantastic. It was great to learn, share, and grow from having her live with us for four weeks.

Retirement

If you have been living a wellness lifestyle all of your life, I am sure that you have been also preparing for the thoughts of retiring. Retiring from work does not mean retiring from wellness. Your career has been holding up your wellness wheel all of these years, and if this spoke is not replaced, you will be out of balance, and you know what that means. It means that it is easier to fall and get hurt. Whatever you do in retirement to replace this spoke, just make sure it is wellness promoting.

There is no better example of how we were built to work, then when a person retires from their career. This is why many seniors take up volunteering in retirement. It is also why some people never fully retire at all. I have heard senior citizens say things like, "After taking vacations, cruises, and playing golf for one year, although these are all fun, I realize how much I miss working." If you have been making plenty of time for leisure throughout life, then you would not feel the overwhelming urge to retire so you can finally relax. Optimally, retirement would be eased into, with the appropriate use of substitutes. (See chapter ten on change.)

Your mind/body needs challenges and events to look forward to, just as much as when you were younger. Studies done on nursing home residents show that when they are given regular challenges and duties, they perform much higher on mind/body tests than the residents that have no responsibilities. No one plans on living in a nursing home, but somebody is ending up there, that's for sure.

This society needs the wisdom that seniors possess. And it is very difficult to share this wisdom while living in an old folks home. Do not let anyone tell you-- "You are too old to do anything productive." Staying active and on a wellness path, increases your odds of staying out of a nursing home.

A car was built to drive, and if you don't ever take it out of the driveway, it will rust and breakdown much faster than if you used it daily. The same principle applies to humans. If we were built to perform meaningful activities, but we don't, then you know what will happen. What will happen is that you will rust away in a smelly building.

Your career, school, and volunteering have to be included when looking at your health status, because spending at least 1/4 of your life-time in these areas absolutely plays a part in your wellness balance. Please keep in mind all of the information we have covered thus far as we complete the wellness circle with the body/mind.

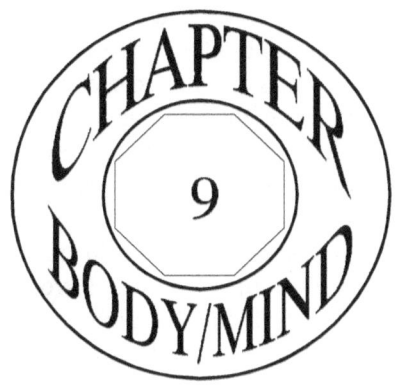

CHAPTER 9
BODY/MIND

I decided to discuss this wellness topic last, for a specific reason. I am sure by now we are getting used to seeing the terms mind and body used as if they were the same word with the same meaning. I chose to use theses terms in various combinations as a way of suggesting that it is the same thing no matter how you say it. Our culture is a little slow to catch onto this concept of body/mind, but the important thing is that it is indeed catching on. I think sometime in the 21st century all literature and people will use these two words, and hopefully understand them to be one and the same.

The body and mind are usually what people will tend to picture when the word wellness is mentioned. However, the bodymind is simply where wellness shows its face. The bodymind perceives, interprets, expresses, and stores wellness. Just because you have no significant dis-eases right now, does not mean that you do not have to worry about your body/mind. I might ask you, "How is your health?" and you claim feeling as healthy as a horse because you only get a cold twice a year. However, if you failed to mention that you are distraught about losing your job, you are sleeping poorly since your separation from your spouse, and your shoulder has been showing signs of arthritis, etc., I know that you are not looking at the big picture. I know plenty of people who claimed to be as healthy as a horse the day before they had a heart attack, and the week before they were diagnosed with cancer. These major dis-eases do not happen at random overnight. They have been in the making for several years. Several years of a not so wellness lifestyle.

One way to look at it is that if your scores of the other seven wellness areas were all rated nines, what score do you think the bodymind area would be? I would have to assume your mindbody rating would also have to be at, or very close to, a score of nine. And if you gave yourself a nine rating across the board and a bodymind rating of a two, I would wonder if you were in your right mind in the first place. Just kidding. Remember any rating you give yourself is perfect because that's how you feel. And your feelings are attached to your emotional molecules, which is what we will now prepare to absorb.

Body/Mind Shift

It is beyond the scope of this book to go into metaphysics and biochemistry, but I will briefly try to describe the body/mind in layman's terms. If you want to understand it in more technical terms, I suggest you find a book called *Molecules of Emotion,* by Candace Pert Ph.D. She is a very famous and fascinating woman in the field of bodymind science.

In her book she describes how emotions are stored in cells throughout the body, and how we are all actually a bunch of vibrating fields of energy. She also states the benefits of touch and its affect on the molecules of emotion. Knowing these principles, I would have to refer you to the therapeutic intervention of Reiki, which is an ancient method of hands-on energy work. Reiki cannot harm in any way, and the benefits can be surprising. It would also follow that the method of massage, especially vibrational massage therapy, produces reports of people laughing and crying during this form of massage, as a result of the release of stored emotions.

We are all aware of how listening to different kinds of music can take us back to emotional episodes of love and sadness, so it would make sense to utilize music for achieving emotional harmony. Don Campbell shows in his resonating book *The Mozart Effect,* how different types of music can influence our emotions. Whenever I listen to my favorite musical artist, Ziggy Marley and the Melody Makers, I immediately have feelings of joy and inspiration, which is typical of reggae music, according to Campbell.

I know that combining body and mind is not an easy shift in thinking. The traditional Western sciences have taught us what we have grown up supposedly knowing, that the body is your bones and skin etc., and your mind is in your brain, and each system does their own thing without interacting with the other systems. We have been taught that our brain carries out its functions independently of the mindbody. Your brain thinks of an action and then it sends messages to the body parts to carry out that action, like tapping your finger. If the new belief is that the mind is non-localized, then that means the mind is everywhere. The mind is in my tapping finger, in my brain, and in my big toe. The mind is in the autonomic nervous system as well as the hairs on my head.

The one example commonly given to explain the body/mind relationship, is that when you have a "gut feeling," you can take this phrase literally. The same thoughts and chemical changes you have in your brain, are also occurring in the cells of your gut--your stomach area. This is not speculation, it is known to be true.

This body/mind concept is difficult to grasp because we cannot see this relationship with our eyes. Astronauts from space cannot see the billions of cars and people bustling around the earth, but we are still here. To the naked eye, the world looks flat but it is not. Our cells are constantly vibrating and changing all over the place, even though we can't see it happening.

We cannot blame ourselves for wanting the mind to be in the head, it seems very logical indeed. This is only because the head is where most of our senses are revealed, but not all. Our eyes, ears, nose, and mouth are all close to the brain. These are simply places where interpretation and expression occurs. A deaf person talks with her hands and fingers, does that mean her mind is in her hands? Yes, actually, it does.

The most powerful idea that Candace Pert presents in her book is:

If it is true that wherever a thought goes -- a chemical goes, then is a chemical a part of the body or the mind, or both?

Although I do believe in the bodymind relationship, I definitely do not have a certain handle on it, but that is alright, as I will keep processing this notion daily. Actually, I have been processing it for years, and now I am adding the spirit into the mix, to confuse the issue even further. This can be a huge undertaking, but I am having a blast with it. I am sure this concept will be much easier for the children of tomorrow to grasp.

If you are wondering whether to buy into this mindbody concept, ask yourself these questions first:

Will it benefit me to know that these two words, body and mind, are really the same thing?

Will it provide for a more clear and deeper insight into my wellness?

Will it allow for healing to occur, if I realize the connection between my chronic pain and the thoughts and emotions I repeatedly have?

Will combining these two concepts, into one, allow me to take more responsibility for my health?

In her book *You Can Heal Your Life*, Louise Hay suggests our physical complaints have a direct connection to our emotions and thoughts. For instance, you may have hearing problems because you are avoiding messages from loved ones or from your intuition. Years ago I would have quickly discounted this theory. However, now knowing how my molecules of emotion work, I am exploring this as a reasonable hypothesis.

Education and Healing

Technically the area of health education could be discussed for infinite pages. Just go to the book store and you will be overwhelmed with the amount of authors helping people overcome specific bodymind dis-eases. Surely you do not have to read them all. Try picking up one of them. It may not be as exhilarating as a romantic suspense thriller, but if you start to take better care of your bodymind now, maybe you will have more time and energy to read more of your favorites for a long time to come. There is no need to feel overwhelmed with bodymind topics, as some books are very easy to comprehend. Even if you only understood half of it, at least you are half way toward increased wellness.

The books I would start most people off with are *Natural Health, Natural Medicine* or *Spontaneous Healing*, by Andrew Weil, M.D. In these books, Dr. Weil informs us of how our mindbody wants a state of balance and peace, and how it is already programmed to do this. Dr. Weil is a Harvard trained, very experienced, and world traveled physician. He is simply interested in helping people to attain homeostasis, and he does not care if that means having surgery, taking herbs, or undergoing hypnosis.

Wellness should not cost you thousands of dollars. Go to the public library and read all you want, for free. The truth is that I never really enjoyed reading, until I started to read topics I personally chose. I recently waited nine months to borrow the highly demanded *Mega Speed Reading*, by Howard Berg, from the library. It was well worth the wait. This is no infomercial gimmick. The techniques are very simple to learn and apply. Since taking this easy course, I have tremendously increased my reading speed and comprehension. Reading is no longer boring because I can read three books in the same time that I used to read one. I would recommend this course to **everyone**, in order to coax you into reading more about wellness topics.

Another tip I want to share, is to buy a compact disc at the music store that only contains instrumental Baroque music. I have been listening to Baroque music while reading, softly in the background, for several years. It works amazingly well to help me focus on the material, while drowning out all extraneous environmental stimuli. The idea is that this specific type of music allows the brain waves on the left and right hemispheres to balance out, which leads to better concentration and retention. It will probably only cost $5 and it can only help. Mozart music can also have the same effects.

Speaking of music, I cannot refrain from mentioning *Sound Body, Sound Mind*, also by Dr.Weil. This instrumental music was specifically designed to promote healing through the arrangement of various frequencies. The music is intended to induce your brain waves into a healing mode. I find this music extremely beautiful and peaceful to my soul. I couldn't tell you if it was actually healing anything, but as long as the intention is there, I never pass up on the chance to experience a placebo response.

Today is the time to start increasing your health education, not tomorrow. Because tomorrow you may be laid up flat on your back in all sorts of pain and confusion for whatever reason, and you will not be able to learn about your health in this compromising situation. You will have to give over your power to others, and apathy does not lead to wellness!

Two years ago, my twenty-two-year-old brother's appendix ruptured, and he had to have it immediately removed. I was surprised to find out the other day that he never did any research, after the fact, as to find out why his appendix may have ruptured. He merely bought into the doctor's explanation that "Sometimes young men have their appendix burst," as if it was a fluke of nature. And we are taught that we really do not need the appendix anyway. Well maybe it was a fluke, or maybe there are various explanations that could also be responsible for the rupture. And if we did not need this body part, then why did God give it to us in the first place?

If one of my body parts broke down so badly that it needed to be removed from my body, you can bet your bottom dollar I am going to do everything in my power to make sure no one else takes out another body part again.(At least until I die, because I am donating my body to science.) How many body parts need to be removed, and how many surgeries does a person need to go through before they start to get educated on body/mind health? My brother is on the honor roll in college and knows how to access information that would help him understand how the appendix works and how it might break down, and how it could have even killed him. Then why doesn't he listen as God/intuition so blatantly screams at him to explore his health?

Maybe he is like the wise man in the flood who let all of his rescuers pass him by.

Educate yourself, because in this era, your physician usually only has enough time to write an illegible prescription, much less, to find out who you really are. I once attended a follow-up visit with my wife to see her ob-gyn, an appointment he requested. After waiting in the examining room for forty-five minutes, he finally came by, giving what was his attempt at a greeting, but I couldn't tell for sure. I am not kidding when I say that this middle aged, smile-less, overweight, Japanese macho doctor had one foot holding open the door while he leaned over toward Dori, who was sitting in a chair near the door, and put the stethoscope on her chest and listened for one breath, asked how she was doing, and then left saying "That's all for now," which concluded the exam. Less than one minute total. And he still had the audacity to bill for this visit and ask for a co-payment. To this day, I never paid this $7 co-payment. Would you pay anyone for any service in which they did not do anything? Unfortunately, I understand that many of us have similar displeasing stories like this one.

If you have a physician who spends all the time you need answering questions and learning about the real you(not the disease you), hold onto this person dearly and send all your friends to him/her.

I am not anti-doctors, although I realize I may come across as such. Allopathic doctors are absolutely needed in the medical field. Many doctors wish they could spend more time on wellness and learning about you, however, there are many constraints built into our current medical system that makes it difficult for them to do so. They are all very well educated. The problem is that most do not have a *diverse* wellness education. A majority of them have been trained at dogmatic universities and hospitals. It is the doctors who have used their intuition, like all the doctors I have mentioned in this book, that see the big picture of body/mind health. These are the modern day Western pioneers who are helping to positively shape our health care system of the next century. God bless them all.

Compliments to Wellness

We can only seek out assistance for healing, from what we are familiar with. If you have no clue what a Doctor of Osteopathy is trained to do, then you would not know that he can greatly improve your state of health after a traumatic accident. It is understandable that you would be reluctant to see an acupuncturist if you did not know anyone that has utilized this modality. But if you knew acupuncture has been practiced by Chinese healers for thousands of years in order to return your chi to a balanced state, and if you knew this brief intervention can only help and cannot do harm, you would feel more at ease when searching for an alternative to things like pain medication or high amounts of anesthesia. And giving it no credence at all does not make sense because it has lasted thousands of years for a reason. If acupuncture had no benefits, the Chinese would have stopped using it long ago.

Assuming there is a formula to healing and that each of us may have a different formula, it would be much more challenging for your intuition to make well informed choices if you were not exposed to the many forms of healing from around the world. I own a book titled *Alternative Medicine*, by the Burton Goldberg Group, which is a compilation of forty different therapies that people can utilize to compliment their wellness circle. Various methods include sound therapy to reduce stress, light therapy to improve your mood, and aroma therapy to treat skin disorders and various infections.

These therapies are intended to compliment allopathic medicine and vice versa. As you know by now, wellness has many parts that have been brought together to create a synergistic formula for healing. The main point is that if you have compromised health, why wouldn't you want to do *whatever* it takes to regain that health? This is why self-education is so important.

Stress

Almost everyone that knows me would tell you that I am a pretty laid-back guy, and that I walk like an old man who doesn't have a care in the world. I consider this to be a compliment, even when it is not their intention. Everyone is affected by stress. I thought that I did not have much stress in my life, but that was before I took a stress management course.(This class was my favorite while in college.) By learning about stress, eustress and distress, I was able to bring more insight to my mindbody. If you have never explored this topic, now would be good. Information on stress management is all over the place and can only benefit you. **No distress = No pain**.

Basically you have to find out where distress manifests in your mind/body. Perhaps it shows up in; your knotted upper trapezius, your clenched fists, your upset stomach, yelling at your kids, spasms in your eyelid, acts of violence, or perhaps a tight lower lip.(Which is where my unmanaged stress shows its face.) After you decide where stress shows up, you will have to discern what preceded it. A bad day at work, an unhappy relationship, or racing thoughts of negativity are a few examples of what can cause unwanted distress. After discovering where it manifests in you and what caused it, there are two choices. You could either prevent the cause, or you could incorporate ways to manage the stress once it arrives. The truth is that you need to do both. Decreasing the causes of distress lessens the amount of stress you have to manage. Unmanaged distress is the opposite of wellness.

Having control of your thoughts is a key factor in regard to this topic. This is evident because whether or not a certain situation is considered to be stressful is up to the individual. Some people love to work with kids, it brings them joy and fulfillment. Other people start to pull their hair out and get very nervous in the presence of active kids. It is not the situation that causes stress, it is the interpreter of the situation that causes stress. So learning how to have greater control over your thoughts and beliefs will have a huge impact on the stress in your life.

Breathwork and meditation are suburb means to control the chatter in your head, which in turn will help to manage stress. These concepts are not mystical, they are practical and highly effective. Both of these techniques are free, and you can engage in them anywhere and anytime. You do not have to move to the Himalaya's or to a monastery to take full advantage breathwork or meditation. The funny thing is that you have been using these tools since birth, but not necessarily in a controlled manner.

Losing a job or having a loved one die unexpectedly can create huge amounts of stress. Last year my company had to down-size due to cutbacks in the Medicare budget. I remember sitting down with my bosses in the office as I calmly listened to the companies regret for having to terminate my position. My pulse and breathing rate increased slightly for about five seconds and then returned to normal. I was honestly not phased by this event. The truth is that my boss was the one who was upset as she did not enjoy having to let me go. Although this would be financially inconvenient, I smiled and new that it was time for me to move on and to have new experiences. Because I know that everything happens for a reason, losing my job was not the stressful event it might have been for someone with no stress management principles. Moving away from this job allowed me the opportunity to follow my true bliss, which is of course, wellness.

Sliding the Wrong Way

When I was twenty-two years old, I played in a slow pitch co-ed softball league during the summer. I was sliding back into first base and twisted my knee. It actually locked up and I couldn't straighten my leg. Somehow my knee slowly "unlocked" and I continued to play. "Call in for a sub, take a break," is what I heard from several of my teammates.

"I'm cool, don't worry," I replied with a painful shriek.

I then proceeded to ungracefully slide into second base on the next play. Again, my knee locked up, except this time it did

86

not "unlock" and I had to be carried off the field. This was a piercing example of how you can make your instinct very mad at you when you do not listen the first time.

This was a very painful injury, more painful than anything I had ever experienced. The first week I was on crutches. I spent most of my time being miserable on the "Lazy Boy" chair, screaming for somebody to get me some ice for the tremendous swelling. I soon went to see two different and very experienced orthopedic surgeons. Both of these physical examinations concluded that it was probably a torn meniscus, which is the cartilage that acts like a shock absorber between the tibia and femur. Both doctors recommended surgery ASAP. Well, what else did I think they would want to do. They are surgeons and that's what they do, surgery.

I was not afraid of needles, operating rooms, and things like this, but I knew surgery was not the answer I was searching for. I thought about it for a week or so, when my minds-eye started to say, "Hey Jim, aren't you studying to become a therapist? Isn't there something you can do to heal our knee?" So I decided to come up with my own prescription for healing.

The starting point after two weeks was a very stiff leg with minimal range of motion, a regular pain level of 5/10 at rest and 8/10 during weight bearing(10/10 would mean the worst pain imaginable), and the swelling around the knee was evident. The first thing I did (which I thought to be totally unrelated at the time) was to read *Diet for a New America*. I picked this book because of a recommendation made by a Tony Robbins(no relation to John)in an audio tape series he has titled *Living Health*. It was summer, and I had nothing else to do but sit in pain and watch television, so I got the book from the library and read it. This was the first book I ever read on my own volition, and not because it was assigned to me as a part of a school course. This book changed my life and absolutely had a huge affect on my healing. I mean to say, the healing of my knee and my entire mindbody.

I belonged to a fitness club, so I took advantage of the swimming pool, sauna, hot tub, and steam room. The pool was perfect for learning how to walk without a limp and for increasing range of motion. The hot tub jets massaged my knee and got the blood flowing to bring nutrients to the damaged tissues. The sauna and steam room allowed me to relax and practice deep breathing to help alleviate the pain. And in there, I physically massaged the edema to push the fluid out of the knee region. I also borrowed an audio tape on visualization which concentrated on self-healing. I practiced the technique of creating little scenarios like having "Super Mario" go to my meniscus and use all of his tools to repair the damage.

The combination of these methods produced amazing results. Within one month I was 60% better, and within three months I was 90% of my old self. I say 90% because before the injury I had hopes of becoming a body builder, but I knew the knee would not be able to easily handle the large amounts of weight needed to create huge muscles. Deep down I new that being a body builder was not in the cards. Lifting weights did produce definite positive results, but I don't think that genetics were in my favor and the desire was gone. Now do not misunderstand, I truly believe I could have been a competitive body builder, but I was not willing to make the sacrifices needed to do so.

I did have my knee lock up two more times within the next two years, from stretching my leg in an awkward position, but it quickly unlocked within a day or so, and I learned how to properly avoid positions that might lead to the knee locking up again. It has been four years since it has locked up and I have no pain, no swelling, and normal range of motion. Of course I do not slide into bases anymore, I only slide forward along my wellness paths.

Unthinkable Healing

Many of us have had these sort of life changing events, such as the situation with my knee. Some choose to learn from these events and grow from them, and some choose to play the victim role and give up. If I could heal myself from a cold, a cough, a fever, and a flu, then why not my knee. We have all overcome these common illnesses, or you would not be reading this book right now. "Those are easy illnesses to beat," Mr. Naysayer might shout from the balcony. If you can beat these common illnesses, then why can't you do the unthinkable, like beating cancer or AIDS.

It wasn't until the 1980's when Dr. Dean Ornish did what his peers deemed to be unthinkable, which was to reverse heart disease without the use of drugs or surgery. Today this is common thinking among his peers. And yes, Mr. Naysayer, there is undeniable proof that people have cured themselves from cancer and AIDS. Which means that we all have this power. We simply need to learn how to access this power. Education in the form of our intuition, a friend, or a book cannot hurt and can only teach us about the unlimited healing ability of the mindbody!

Take for instance, Earvin "Magic" Johnson. I remember several years ago feeling shocked when it was announced that he was HIV positive. As of this writing, Mr. Johnson is very healthy, and is an extremely successful businessman. I predicted from the beginning that Magic would not be afflicted with AIDS, he would live a long life, and would only die from natural causes. Mainly because he stopped engaging in a dangerous lifestyle and he began to build his wellness. He did not play the victim role, he became proactive.

If you can overcome a cold, which is a virus, then why can't you overcome HIV, which is, of course, a virus? (A virus so minute that blood tests can only find the antibodies for HIV, and not HIV itself.) I know this sounds simplistic, but maybe it is real. Furthermore, there is a book written by Peter Duesberg titled *Inventing the AIDS Virus*, in which he reveals that HIV has never been proven to cause AIDS. I strongly suggest to anyone who is HIV positive, to read this book to obtain an alternate view on this highly political subject. I am not making any recommendations, because I could get in trouble, however, I can say that if I were to be somehow diagnosed as being positive for HIV, I would not take any prescription drugs. I would simply continue my course of high level wellness. Because it is not HIV that kills people, it is their lack of a wellness lifestyle that kills them.

I would also like to recommend a book called *Remarkable*

Recovery, by Hirshberg & Barasch, to everyone, and especially those diagnosed with cancer. This book suggests there is a *formula* to healing yourself from anything, and that the *formula* is <u>unique</u> to your bodymind. That is why getting in-tune with your intuition is so important. If you were in-tune, there is a good chance you wouldn't have become ill in the first place. But in the chance that you do become ill, it is your intuition that will also lead you to recovery.

Part of Norman Cousins' formula for healing was laughter. It seemed ridiculous to believe that watching hours worth of "Abbott and Costello" comedy classics would have such a positive impact on his life threatening illness. Mr.Cousins listened to the knower inside who knew laughter would bring his molecules of emotion to the right places for healing to occur. Laughter was a huge part of his healing formula.

Anecdotal evidence of healing formulas are usually discounted by science. If it cannot be proven by clinical research then it cannot be given any credence. If I were someone in desperate need of healing, I am not going to wait around for science to get around to discovering my formula for healing through clinical trials. I will use my intuition to reveal the factors that may be unique to my formula for healing, whether that means laughter, getting closer to my spirituality, drinking carrot juice, or listening to someone's anecdotal healing experiences. The only formula that counts is the one that works!!!

If one of the main reasons a person can get cancer is due to an inefficient immune system, then why would it make sense to bombard a person with toxic chemicals that weaken the immune system even further. Ask your doctor to see the clinical studies that prove what he proposes you go through, to be more effective than doing something else or even doing nothing at all. You may be surprised to find out that going through dangerous treatments may actually show not to be more effective than other alternatives. And if this doctor refuses to provide you with the evidence, then go see another doctor that will.

I know this sounds absurd, why would a doctor recommend something that does not prove to be the only option. Like I said before, if you go to a surgeon he will want to do surgery. If you go to a produce market for nutrition, the workers will want to sell you fruits and vegetables, but if you go to a butcher, guess what he will try to sell you! If you only go to an oncologist for cancer treatment recommendations, guess what he/she is going to sell you on? I predict that fifty-years from now we will see things like chemotherapy and radiation therapy to be highly barbaric.

A final thought on education. I foresee a day when wellness will be taught from preschool to high school graduation. Questions on worksheets will ask how to figure out the proper daily required sleep fraction. I also foresee the day when exact history dates of small battles are less important than learning about the history of bodymind medicine. A day when you can say the word *God* in public schools without being expelled. You can see where I am going with this. Yes, learning how to use a computer and all this modern technology "stuff" is important, but I would rather have my child first know the foundation for pure health, happiness, and longevity. The rest is gravy.

Thoughts

If you are the kind of person who feels you cannot control your thoughts, I hate to be the bearer of bad news, but the truth is that only you control your thoughts. You are not a puppet, you are a human. God blessed you with the gift of thoughts. He also gave you the gift of choice. A phrase Wayne Dyer often uses is, "You become what you think about all day long." If there is anything you can learn from this program, understand that phrase. If throughout the day, you keep telling yourself, "I am so tired and stressed out, and I do not have the energy to do anything," then you won't have the energy.

"Argue for your limitations and they are yours."

"He who expects nothing out of life will not be disappointed."

I could give a million examples of various thought limiting and thought promoting scenarios, but you are intelligent enough to understand this principle.

I read a book called *What to Say When You Talk to Yourself,* by Dr. Shad Helmstetter, which reveals how what we tell ourselves(self-talk)will have a direct impact on our bodymind health. Remember, wherever a thought goes--a chemical goes. So if your thoughts are going to a place that says you are a failure and that you would be better off dead, guess where your chemicals are going? They are going to find a way to help you achieve your thoughts of destruction. If your thoughts want balance, and if your self-talk keeps repeating, "I am building my wellness circle and I am getting stronger each day," then your chemicals will find a way to make this a reality. In other words, self-fulfilling prophecies are real. As you think, so shall you be.

When thoughts come, that you do not want, simply acknowledge them, thank them for coming, then ask them to close the door on their way out. Yes, the thought may come back periodically, but eventually it will get the hint and perhaps it will stop coming all together. With time and practice these thoughts will simply send you a postcard once a year, and eventually they will die or lose your address. Sometimes when I catch myself following thoughts that do not benefit me, I will literally yell out STOP! This breaks the thought pattern in an instant. Then I say aloud, "think positive." Try it, it works for me.

Most situations we think to be major problems are actually self-created. We can only live one day at a time. Have you ever heard the saying, "Live one yesterday at a time" or "Live one tomorrow at a time?" Of course not. Thoughts of guilt = living in the past, and thoughts of worry = living in the future. The amazing fact is that we have sixty-thousand thoughts each day, but even more amazing is that they were probably the same thoughts we had the day before, and the day before that.

What you choose to focus your thoughts on *will* have an enormous impact on your wellness. If we have negative thoughts today, the odds are that we will continue to have them over and over. So why would you have thoughts that do not benefit you? For me, just knowing that experiencing happiness is my core reason for being here on earth, gives me better insight into my own thoughts. Your thoughts are actually the key component to all of the other wellness areas. If you cannot control your thoughts, it would be impossible to have control of your wellness.

The best selling *Your Erroneous Zones*, will give you tremendous understanding into the art of taking control of your thoughts and feelings, and in my opinion, should be standard reading in all high schools. If everyone read and understood the words Wayne Dyer put in this book, many therapists would be out of work. Also, focused meditation will lead to firmer control of your thoughts.

In *Health and Healing*, Dr.Weil explores the phenomenon of the placebo effect, which he prefers to call the placebo response. The term placebo response is more accurate because if it truly was a placebo, how could it have had an *effect* on anything. The truth is that your mindbody had a *response* to the placebo.

In the end it almost seems like our beliefs are at the core of healing. First of all, you had to believe enough to find the specific practitioner or healer. Next, you had to believe, somewhat at least, what the person prescribed for you might help. Finally, you had to believe whether or not the intervention actually made a difference or not. Who knows, maybe some day we will all be healed by sugar pills for any dis-ease you can imagine.

I am not so naive to suggest that life is only peaches and cream. We are all guaranteed to experience very unpleasant events in life, some we can prevent and some are out of our control. Numerous unexpected life occurrences can strike us out of the blue at any time. It is our wellness resources that will determine how we deal with these events. If your wellness ratings were all two's and three's, it is almost certain that you will have a more difficult time overcoming these events, as opposed to having wellness ratings that were all eight's and nine's. Wouldn't you agree?

One wellness thought I have ingrained in me is that everything happens for a reason. There are no accidents or coincidences. The tough part of this thinking is that the reason may not become obvious for a long time. This will teach you patience, and infinite patience produces immediate results, as stated in *A Course in Miracles*.

Crutches

When we experience pain or discomfort, we want to know what is causing it, so we search for a diagnosis. If you go to your physician, she too will search for a diagnosis, partly because that is how doctors get reimbursed. Scientists try to come up with numerous diagnostic categories and codes in order to explain all the possible illnesses in the world. And when a new illness is discovered, like AIDS, it too is given a new code. If something does not fit into a category they have created, for instance if a person has Bipolar disease that doesn't exactly fit into an established code, they say you have Bipolar Disease NOS, or not otherwise specified. These diagnostic codes are extremely important in understanding the course of an illness.

The point I am making is that you are not a code, not a prescription, and not a dis-ease. You are a whole person. Complicated maybe, but definitely whole. Do not get attached to any diagnosis that someone has labeled you with. People with cancer are never considered to be cured from this illness, they are merely considered to be in "remission." The term remission does little for a person's confidence. If you "catch" a cold, and five days later it is completely gone, does that mean you are in remission, because you will probably catch another cold before you die someday?

Another classic example of labeling is how someone who was once addicted to alcohol, but it has been twenty, thirty, or forty years since they had a drink, and that person has never once been tempted to go back to that lifestyle. Why do some of these people continue to say they are recovering alcoholics? Have you ever heard someone say, who has not had any caffeine beverages for twenty years, that they are recovering caffeineoholics? What's the difference? Aren't they both drugs? I know I will get heat for saying this, but it is what I truly wonder. Why label yourself as anything that is no longer accurate! I do not go around calling myself a recovering agnostic, it is simply something that I no longer identify with.

When I was nine years old, my mother took me and my

brother to a podiatrist to remove what my father coined "Hamburger Feet." What he meant was that we had excessive skin peeling on the bottom of our feet. Anyway, during the routine foot exam, the doctor detected that I had flat feet and recommended I be fitted for orthotic inserts to wear inside my shoes. This would help to mold my foot in order to have an arch over time, like normal kids. Well no one ever asked me if I wanted these uncomfortable, awkward, plastic things in my shoes, and up until this point in life I thought I was normal. But hey, the doctor said so and that was good enough. The only reason I remember being given for having the orthotics was that I needed an arch because the Army did not accept men with flat feet. Like this is a huge concern for a nine-year-old!

I had to go to his office regularly to be casted, fitted and refitted as my foot continued to grow. The tall, overweight, sixty-year-old, Irish doctor would melt the orthotics with a heat gun and minutely increase the arch angle at each visit. He would then watch me walk up and down the hallway and say "Good Jimmy, you're getting better."

"Getting better from what?" was my shrugging thought.

Finally, my foot stopped growing. The doctor took me downstairs and bought me a strawberry milk shake, then told me that this was the end of the road, which can also be interpreted as, "Thanks for the business kid, now beat it."

I eagerly responded, "So what do I do now, can I throw these things away?"

"No," he laughed, "You keep wearing them for the rest of your life."

When I wore the orthotics, which was always, I was uncomfortable for the first few weeks after he refitted them, and eventually I felt no discomfort. But when I walked around the house barefoot, my foot would often start to cramp up. So I naturally assumed that the orthotic was working, because I didn't get cramps when I wore them.

Several years later we got a new dog from the humane society. For some reason this dog loved my orthotics and he chewed one of them up pretty good. At that time I was living in the Big Island of Hawaii and I was only wearing the orthotics to work. When I came home I wore "Slippahs," which is a local saying for sandals. It was so humid that almost no one wore shoes outside of work. So I had been slowly moving away from the orthotics anyway. I pondered repairing the orthotic, but my intuition distinctly told me, as I held this crutch in my hand, to forget about it because I did not need them. I did not need them now, I did not need them when I was nine years old, and I did not need them ever! Needless to say, I have no problems with my feet anymore, and I feel superb.

Why tell this story? How many of you are carrying around an old crutch. Either self-created, or a crutch that was kindly given to you by your doctor. I probably would have worn those things to my grave, if it wasn't for Moku, the island dog.(Moku in Hawaiian means to be set free, which is what we did for him, by freeing him from the pound, and he returned the favor by setting me free of my crutches.) He still routinely chews up many loose things around the house, and Dori always wonders why I never scold him for doing this. She claims I spoil him. How could I ever consider scolding him, when he was the angel who gave me back my feet!!

Maybe your crutch is your eye glasses that you were told you needed because you couldn't read a letter on a chart one day. Maybe your crutch is the anxiety medication and diagnosis your doctor gave you during a time of intense anxieties. And now you always feel you need the drug to prevent the possibility of another attack. Although you haven't had an attack for years, you still use the medication as a crutch. Maybe your crutch is the label you were given as a child, labels like "You are just not good at math," or "You are simply a slow reader." Or your crutch may literally be a crutch, and there is still hope. Remember what Forrest Gump did with his crutches? Consider this notion as a possibility to regain your body-mind health.

Now that we have discovered all of the components that lead to wellness for~every~one, it only makes sense that we explore how to make lasting *changes* forever.

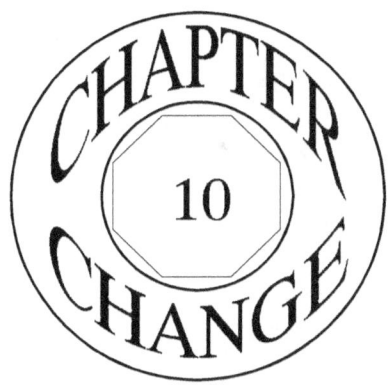

CHAPTER 10 CHANGE

There are many book topics out there that have the word *change* in it, which show you how to make lasting personal changes in your life. Change can be as easy or as difficult as we want it to be. There are only two choices you have in regard to change. You can either change the situation, or you can change the way you approach the situation. It will always be more difficult if you are trying to change someone else without their permission, so move way from this notion right now, it almost never works. When you think of change, think only about yourself. People who make positive changes in their life as a part of a wellness lifestyle will rub off on others. I have come to this knowing through experience.

When I first made major diet modifications in my life, which provided powerful benefits, I was eager to share this fantastic message with everyone, many times in an overzealous fashion. I soon came to discover I could not change anyone else or the world with my enthusiasm, in one day. Now I simply live the way that makes me happy, and others will soon come discover what my message is. And as Mahatma Gandhi simply put it, "My life is my message."

Now people come to me with questions about wellness on their own volition, because they know my message, as opposed to my giving unsolicited advice to my family and friends.

Always Changing

My wife tells me she hates it when I frequently make a positive modification in my wellness lifestyle.

"Why is that?" I asked her one day.

"Because you can simply say something like you will cut back 75% on your salt intake and you will do it, just like that," she says in an irritated manner.

Making frequent changes in your life does not mean you are a hypocrite or a wishy washy person. It is more likely a sign you realize that what you are practicing now is not beneficial. And if it is not benefiting you, why keep doing it? If making a change can only help and cannot hurt, what is the harm in trying it. And if that change does not work, then you can make another change until you get it right.

Making time for wellness does not mean that you have to make hundreds of changes all at once. But you have to start somewhere. Every little change counts. By no means do I think my wellness wheel has stopped growing just because I wrote this book. For instance, my next simple change towards wellness is going to be to finish the last few ice-pops I have in my freezer. And the next time I go shopping, I will search for an ice-pop that does not contain any artificial colors or sweeteners. This change can only help and cannot harm me. It wasn't too radical and it did not take much effort to buy a new frozen treat. It may seem insignificant on the surface, but wellness is ongoing and it is a lot of little things that add up to huge benefits.

Comfort Zones

Last year I purchased a filter for my shower head. I heard how chlorine can contribute to unbalanced skin appearance, which I have been experiencing long past puberty. At first I thought the idea of filtering my shower water was very peculiar. But I will never forget the feeling when the filtered water first touched my skin, it was wonderful. I have definitely seen an improvement in my skin since using this shower filter. (Even when I sit in the Jacuzzi, although I never put my face in the water, my face still breaks-out because the chlorine was absorbed throughout my skin, below my neck.)

It wasn't until three weeks later, when I took a shower at my parents house, that I realized how I felt after taking a shower with chlorinated water for the last decade. The point I am getting at is that what we consider to be normal may not be so normal until we *change*, until we have *new* experiences. Now that I have changed my shower head, I know that unfiltered water was not benefiting me. This same sobering example holds true when most *changes* are made toward wellness and away from "normal."

Often, we get stuck in our comfort zones and convince ourselves that we know what is best for us. But if we never go outside of this comfort zone, we will not get to experience all that life has to offer. I see an example of this comfort zone mentality when I go out to eat with my brother. He is what I consider to be a very picky eater. He limits himself to what and where he will eat. I always want to try out new places to eat lunch, but he is very reluctant because he already knows what the best is, so he usually insists on going to the same places every time. Certainly I have my favorite places to eat also, but I had to go outside my comfort zone in the first place to find this favorite place, and I will have to go outside my current comfort zone in order to find new favorites.

There are many safe ways to start to expand your comfort zones. One thing I do to spontaneously expand my comfort zone mentality is when it is time for a hair cut. I just get in my truck and pull up to a new barber shop every two months. I get to meet a new person and experience new surroundings. I usually walk into the establishment and break the ice by asking, "How much will you charge to make me look like Tom Cruise." I will often get a response of, "Son, it will take more money than you can imagine," and then we will have a good laugh together. Once, I asked that question and the guy said, "I can't make you look like Tom Cruise but I can make you look like Yul Brynner."

Even when I find a barber who actually takes his time and

cuts my hair exactly like I asked him to, I will not hesitate to go to a new barber shop the next time. Making simple non-threatening changes to expand your comfort zones may provide you the confidence to make more important changes in regard to wellness.

Goals

I am surprised I have not thanked Anthony Robbins yet, as he has been a wonderful influence in my life. He has programs on how to make lasting changes in your life, through the premises of NLP(neuro linguistic programming.) If you haven't by now, please get your hands on anything he has created. It can't hurt, that's for sure. He is partly the reason I am here today sharing this message. I remember driving home from school one gorgeous afternoon, listening to Tony, when he said, "If you are in your car, stop the tape, pull over, and do this life defining exercise on goal setting--right now!" My instinct knew not to ignore him, so I immediately pulled over and wrote down my goals. One of my goals has been to become a renowned public speaker, that was always a certainty after doing the exercise that afternoon. What was not certain for many years was what I would talk about.

An acronym that Tony has created, which I have incorporated into my life, is C.A.N.I.=constant and never-ending improvement. This is like the wellness wheel approach, it just keeps getting larger and larger. I am not suggesting that we should not be happy with the way things are right now. Remember, we are perfect exactly how we are right now, and yet we can always choose to further develop our wellness circle.

Through Tony's teachings, I am now several steps closer to achieving all of my long term goals.

I am a strong believer in writing down your goals. In my consulting business, I have my clients physically write down their own goals in each wellness area and then I ask them to say it aloud. I know I said earlier that you would not have to pick up a pencil again while reading this book, and you don't, but it sure could not hurt to write down your wellness goals.

There are two kinds of goals, short term and long term. All major achievements start off with a short term goal before the long term goal is reached. Writing and saying your goals serves a few purposes. It helps to process your thinking. It helps you to actually see the goal, at least on paper. It will help you to commit to the goal because you created it and you said you were going to do it. The goal needs to be reasonable, measurable, and achievable, and should have a time frame.

A common wellness goal may read: "I will fill up a half gallon of water each morning and I will drink it all, throughout the day, for one week." A poorly created goal would read: "I will try to drink more water." How could you measure whether you achieved this goal? Another good wellness goal would read: "I will call my loved one every day at 10:45 AM during my break at work, in order to improve our open communication about sex." A lacking goal would be: "I will call my loved one more often to talk about stuff."

Make it easy on yourself, write down simple and reasonable goals, then build off of them. Writing down long term goals may be more challenging, only because it is hard to set time frames, and what may be realistic in the future may appear impossible today.

Accomplishing long term goals requires you to have a clear vision. My ideas of being a renowned public speaker are certainly against the odds, but it is absolutely possible. And if it is possible, if you have a vision, and you want it passionately enough, then give yourself the chance and write it down, and then say it aloud with confidence.

It is fine if your goals change over time, so if you are hung up with working toward a goal you set years ago but you honestly have no desire to achieve it anymore, then stop wasting your time and set some new goals.

Wellness Goals -Worksheet

All goals need to start with **I will**, as opposed to I'll try or I will not. These goals must also be achievable, measurable, reasonable, and should have a time frame. Take your time and allow your intuition to guide you when writing down these goals. After completing this, post it up on your refrigerator so you will see it every day.

ST=short term goals. LT= long term goals.

Family and Friends
ST: *I will*_____
LT: *I will*_____

Nutrition
ST: *I will*_____
LT: *I will*_____

Sleep
ST: *I will*_____
LT: *I will*_____

Body-Mind
ST: *I will*_____
LT: *I will*_____

Spirituality
ST: *I will*_____
LT: *I will*_____

Leisure
ST: *I will*_____
LT: *I will*_____

Fitness
ST: *I will*_____
LT: *I will*_____

Career
ST: *I will*_____
LT: *I will*_____

Everyone Changes

I listened to an audio cassette recently, titled *Return of the Rishi*, by Dr. Deepak Chopra. I will assume by now most everyone has heard his name, as he is a tremendously respected pioneer in the field of wellness. I was surprised to learn that Deepak was not practicing nearly any of the things he practices and teaches today. For instance, Deepak and his father were trained in, and strictly practiced, allopathic medicine. He did not really pay any mind to the way he lives now, which is an Ayervedic lifestyle. He smoked cigarettes, and drank coffee and alcohol regularly. On top of that, he worked very long hours with little sleep, as an internist.

During one of his many trips back to India from the east coast, his friend took him to see an Ayervedic doctor, who read Deepak's pulse. The doctor told him his life was moving too fast and he needed to slow down. Soon after, Deepak began the practice of meditation, and he reports that although it was not his goal, it was three days later that he realized he had not even had one cigarette. This was the beginning of his wellness journey that he is so gracefully sharing with the world today. So it is humbling to know that he was not born knowing his enlightenment, he had to change and discover it just like the rest of us.

Making wellness lifestyle changes are surely within the grasp of everyone. Sometimes when I tell people about the wellness practices I have, a common reaction is "Wow, that sounds great, but I know I could never be able to _____."(You fill in the blank: sleep that well, eat that well, etc.) I hope they realize, deep down, that their inner self knows the truth. The truth is that neither I, your neighbor, the fitness guy on television, Deepak Chopra, or Tony Robbins are equipped with any magic bullets. We have all been gliding along the wellness path, and it did not happen overnight.

Many of the people I refer you to in this book were not born with a high level of wellness or enlightenment. John Robbins had polio as a child. Dr. John McDougall had a stroke while in college, and still has a limp to this day. Wayne Dyer lived in an orphanage. Tony Robbins and Andrew Weil both reflect on a time in their lives when they were very unhappy and overweight. Candace Pert writes about a time she was in the hospital and remained flat on her back for weeks, highly medicated by morphine to kill the pain caused by a horse back riding incident. Mona Lisa Schultz depicts her bout with narcolepsy and being hit by a truck while running, two weeks after graduating college, resulting in many broken bones and a collapsed lung. And Louise Hay's background is too horrible to describe.

These people are no more gifted than you or I, they have simply chosen to utilize the gifts God gave them. The gifts God has given to all of us.

Believe It

Wayne Dyer has a book called *You'll See it When You Believe it*. You might be thinking I said this backward because the saying usually goes, "I'll believe it when I see it with my own eyes." The former phrase creates a whole new mind shift toward making changes. Actually we do this all the time. We go to college with the belief that we will someday see ourselves working in the field of our choice. We believe that our children will grow up to be fine citizens even before they can walk.

You need to have belief and faith to make your dreams come true. For instance, I believe I am a future national public speaker with a very important message, which folks want to come see and hear. I believed this would be true for many years, even though it actually never happened. And because of my faith, I am getting closer to experiencing this dream, I can see it evolving with my own eyes. I also practice visualization, meaning, I see myself making presentations to audiences all the time, which helps me to believe my goal is possible. Although this goal is not yet a reality, it is my faith that keeps me focused on this goal.

If you want to build a large wellness wheel, it does not have to be a huge undertaking or a struggling effort in change. Maybe you cannot *see* yourself living a wellness lifestyle because you have never experienced a wellness lifestyle. On the contrary, according to the diagram you filled out at the beginning of this book, we are all experiencing some degree of wellness. Otherwise you would be dancing in the clouds somewhere. You are simply not experiencing the high wellness level you desire.

Let's now go through an example of a "You'll see it when you believe it" scenario.

What is your goal? "To be a person who has high level wellness."

Why? "In order to experience all that I am entitled to, which is maximum health, happiness, and longevity."

How do you get to this state of wellness?

Start by closing your eyes, while sitting comfortably in a room, alone. Take four slow deep breaths, and picture yourself in a pleasant place. See yourself experiencing your wellness goals. You are living it in your minds-eye. You are living the lifestyle you desire, and you truly believe it is possible. You are aware of all eight wellness areas, which is your whole life. Do this for as long as the pictures are clear and focused, the longer the more memorable.

Do not forget those images, and if you ever do forget those wellness images, create some that are more vivid and unforgettable. And if no images come right now, keep trying daily because they will come if you give them the opportunity.

How old were you in those images? Where were you? Who was with you? What were you doing? All that you just visualized can be reality, maybe not tomorrow, but that's not the point. As I repeatedly suggest, the main point is that we are moving in the right direction. If you cannot see where you are going, how can you expect to get there and how will you know when you have arrived?

Did you ever have a hand drawn map on how to get to a friends house in a city you have never been to? The start and end point were clear, but the roads that led to the house were all mixed up, and the napkin it was drawn on was getting frayed. Despite all of this, you still managed to find your friend. Maybe your intuition helped you figure out very quickly that Main Street had to be the only way that made sense. Or maybe your rishi told you to stop and ask for directions, that is if your rishi is a woman, of course. Or maybe your inner self told you to call your friend and say, "Come get me, I am lost and I don't want to go around in circles anymore." All answers are correct if you were closely listening to your inner awareness. If you have no vision and you do not ask for help then you might drive around in circles for years and years.

Change comes through seeing and believing and vice versa. It is easier to see and believe any subject you are having challenges with, if you study and practice that subject.

Wellness is your whole life, and I assume we are all studying and practicing life every day. But if you keep reading the same book, thinking the same thoughts, and walking the same walk, change would almost be impossible. So what am I saying? Read a new book, think a new thought, walk a new walk. It doesn't have to be all in the same day. Just take one step at a time, in the right direction, as we have heard a thousand times before. Then slowly watch as your wellness wheel gets bigger and starts to become a giant snowball, except this snowball never ends, it keeps going as long as you want, even beyond this lifetime. All of the authors I have mentioned in this chapter are like snowballs. They just keep getting bigger and bigger and we can't get enough.

Belief Worksheet

Beliefs play a major influence on what your wellness wheel will look like. The following are personal examples of changes in beliefs I have made in each wellness area over the past few years.

Nutrition
Old belief: *Cow's milk is necessary for strong bones, and if I don't drink it daily, I will get osteoporosis.*
Current belief: *Milk is for babies.*

Spirituality
Old belief: *There probably is no such thing as God and there is no life after death.*
Current belief: *God is everywhere and in everything and there is no end to life.*

Career
Old belief: *A large salary with good security is what is most important in a job.*
Current belief: *Flowing with bliss is what is important and it is why I am here to contribute to this world.*

Leisure
Old belief: *Watching football on Sunday is plenty of time for leisure.*
Current belief: *I need both active and passive leisure activities for complete wellness.*

Fitness
Old belief: *More is better, pain is OK, competition is everything.*
Current belief: *Balanced and safe exercise is fun and effective.*

Sleep

Old belief: *I need to watch television before sleeping, or I won't be able to easily fall   asleep.*

Current belief: *I can easily fall asleep after reading a book or listening to relaxing music.*

Body-Mind

Old belief: *My thoughts have nothing to do with my physical health.*

Current belief: *I become what I think about all day long.*

Family-Friends

Old belief: *It is OK if I try to change my loved ones as long as I have good intentions.*

Current belief: *I have no right to try to change others and I love them exactly how they are now.*

Belief Worksheet

I now encourage you to fill out the worksheet to identify your own former and current beliefs in each area. The purpose of this exercise is to allow you to reflect on the powerful effects of your beliefs, and how changes in beliefs have changed your life. Ask yourself why you made those changes. Hopefully your current beliefs are closer to wellness than your old beliefs. I assume your current beliefs have some benefits over the old beliefs. The question you and your intuition need to explore is: Will new beliefs change my wellness circle for the better?

Nutrition

Old belief:_____

Current belief:_____

Spirituality

Old belief:_____

Current belief:_____

Career
Old belief:_____
Current belief:_____

Leisure
Old belief:_____
Current belief:_____

Fitness
Old belief:_____
Current belief:_____

Sleep
Old belief:_____
Current belief:_____

Body-Mind
Old belief:_____
Current belief:_____

Family-Friends
Old belief:_____
Current belief:_____

Substitution

It is often much easier to make changes if you have a substitute for whatever it is you are moving away from. That is what change is all about, moving away from this behavior or that line of thinking, and hopefully moving toward a wellness type of behavior and thought process. The problem many people encounter is that they know what to move away from, but they do not know what to move toward. It is more beneficial to think in terms of moving away from and moving toward, as opposed to quitting and starting.

The word quitting is associated with negative feelings, it makes you feel like what you were doing was wrong or bad. And what happens if you cannot quit (whichever behavior or thoughts you choose) cold turkey? Then you might feel as if you failed and couldn't do it. Moving toward wellness gives you much more leeway and much more opportunity to grow and problem solve. Whatever you are moving away from, it most likely served a purpose. The tricky part sometimes is being able to find out what the purpose was. If you always bit your nails for twenty years, and then you decided to move away from this, you would have to discover what the purpose was for biting them in the first place. Only then will you know what you need to move toward. If biting your nails was a nervous habit related to being alone, then you would have to find another way to manage the feelings of being alone.(Or maybe you just need to move toward a drug store and buy some nail clippers.) Yes we are creatures of habit, but these habits probably serve some kind of purpose.

Nutrition is probably the easiest way to understand the substitution principle. Many people cannot fathom the thought of moving away from hamburgers, but their doctor just told them how dangerously high their cholesterol and triglyceride levels were. You would think this alone would scare a person to quit eating hamburgers. But it often does not work, because quitting anything cold turkey is difficult, and the person has not yet had the opportunity to find a suitable replacement. I suggest to slowly integrate substituting meat burgers with the very tasty and readily available "veggie" burger or "garden" burger. The next time you have meatloaf, simply mix in half hamburger and half veggie burger, and then slowly taper the amount over time until it is all "veggieloaf." Now you have something to move away from and something to move toward. This move may happen in one day or maybe in one month, but as long as you are moving in the right direction, the substitution is working!

Substitutes do not have to be a sacrifice. Your eating habits are a learned behavior. If you grew up in Mexico, you would have learned to love the taste of rice, beans, and tortillas. If you were from Italy, you would have learned to love the taste of pasta and vegetables. If you learned to like a hamburger, you can learn to like a veggie burger. If you learned to like the taste of cow's milk, you can learn to like the taste of rice milk, soy milk, or almond milk. (My favorite is chocolate almond milk, which I pour over my cereal.) If you learned to like the taste of coffee, you can learn to like the taste of herbal teas. I have never met a baby who was born with cravings for coffee.

I assume that no one reading this book considers themselves unable to learn, or you would not be reading it in the first place. Making nutritional substitutions are easy once you know the formula.

This formula can work the same way for all of the wellness areas. We already covered how to slowly substitute your current career with the career your bliss desires. Let's try a hard one in the family wellness area. Let's say you wanted to move away from criticizing your spouse, an unproductive habit which usually gets you nowhere. We have to ask what purpose was being served by constantly criticizing your spouse. Maybe you do it as a means of retaliation because they supposedly started in on you first. Maybe you do it because when you were a kid everyone in your household found faults in each other when they were mad. Maybe you criticize your spouse because you feel the life they are living is unhealthy, and you are being selfish by wanting them to be around with you for a long time.

Once you discover why you are behaving and thinking this way, how do you quit? Ah ha, remember, completely quitting something like this, cold turkey, is almost impossible. We have to now decide that criticizing others is usually not beneficial or nice. Lastly, we have to find a substitute for this habit. So the next time you feel like saying "You are a slob, the house is a mess," you can pause and say, "Hunny I love you very much, you are a wonderful person." Try saying this too if you are on the receiving end of an unpleasant criticism. This does not mean that you should avoid stating your wishes, on the contrary, you should always let your wishes be known. However, if you have already made your wishes known in the form of criticism one hundred times before, the one hundred and first probably will not make a difference.

Another option would be to know that criticizing does not bring happiness, and what you really want is for the house to be clean anyway, so simply clean it yourself, even if you didn't make the mess. The act of cleaning up may not bring you pleasure, but a clean, criticize-free home will bring you happiness. And then you will have more time for love and less time for stress.

Mentors

Changes are easier to make when you are inspired by a mentor. I think toddlers can be great examples of a mentor for wellness. Although it sounds bizarre, let me make my case. Toddlers have excellent posture. They do not complain of back pain and they do not need the back of a chair to sit upright. Toddlers release their toxic wastes when they need to, in order to prevent this toxic waste from backing up into their system. They eat when their tummies are hungry, not when their eyes are hungry. They sleep when they are tired and they wake up when they are fully rested, not when the alarm clock tells them they are rested. Toddlers smile freely and are very spontaneous. Both boys and girls ask for hugs with ease, and they do not hold in emotions. Work and fitness is their play. They adapt to change easily. These amazing creatures do not worry about yesterday or tomorrow, they only focus on the present moment. These perfect beings do not have complexes about being pretty enough or skinny enough, and they have no shame about their bodies. They will listen to any opinions on spirituality with openness and without bias. Their instinct/God guides them when they are ready to walk, and when they fall, they get right back up without hesitation.

This all sounds like an excellent wellness mentor to me. What do you think?

If your brother is an expert on fitness, then do what he does. If your mother is a super healthy eater, then eat like she does. If your friend is a happy family man, then ask him what his principles are in regard to family happiness. Do you get the picture? The old saying, "You do not have to reinvent the wheel," suggests that we are supposed to learn from others. Wellness leaves clues, so all you have to do is follow the trail. Take the time to study success, but first take the time to study the next chapter on time.

CHAPTER 11

TIME

"Jim, how can I possibly do all of these wellness things, it all sounds good, but I don't have the time, it doesn't fit into my schedule."

"Oh yea, just let me know who creates your schedule and I'll have a talk with them."

I hear this saying every day, sometimes from my own mouth. Most likely, the fact is not that you do not have the time for wellness, it is that you <u>choose</u> not make the time.

I am not insensitive to this challenge, I face it every day just like you. However, I think finding ways to make time for wellness is easier than you may choose to think. The simplest way I know how, would be to combine wellness areas together. For example, here is a three for one deal. Your favorite leisure activity of all time is bicycling, the fresh out-door air, the speed, the freedom, you love it. It also happens to fulfill the wellness area of fitness, assuming you don't only ride downhill. You can also incorporate the wellness area of spending more time with your family and friends, so you go riding with your kid, spouse, or neighbor.

Here is another three for one deal. Your favorite leisure activity is your love of cooking. It allows for creativity, and time flies by. Simply invite someone to join you, or teach your kids.

They love to help make meals, and you are also focusing on your nutrition area. One more three for one bargain. You love to go for long drives as a leisure activity, and you listen to spirituality related audio cassettes at the same time with your family, or career related cassettes, with your friend.

Two for one deals are also readily on sale. The most common one I can think of are business lunches. Eating meals together is one of the first social events we experience as children and throughout evolution, it is a natural event. So don't eat alone if you can help it. Falling asleep each night in the arms of your spouse, or reading a nightly story to your child, are easy and fun ways to improve your wellness.

The road block you may have about making enough time can lie in the way you look at each area or the way others look at the areas. I really despised my long commute from Daly City to San Jose State University twice a week. To me this was a waste of time, and I would always get pains in my back from excessive periods of sitting in the car and in classes. I did not think pleasantly about spending time doing this at all.

Now, driving is a different story. Why? Because I took steps toward changing various factors. This is when I discovered books on tape, which I still listen to regularly. This made traveling more interesting than listening to the same songs and flipping through commercials for the one hour drive. And I loved the idea of learning new things, at least I was using this time productively. Around the same time, I went to see a chiropractor who helped to relieve my back pain through adjustments, and he showed me a few exercises to lessen and prevent the back pain, which all worked nicely. I also took a stress management class which taught meditation and breathwork, which I practiced on the drive home after a long day, to prevent muscle and mind tension. Today, I always look forward to long drives if I have my tapes to listen to. So the idea is that a shift in approach allowed for enjoyment of driving and gave me time to improve my body/mind, as these were usually the kinds of tapes I listened to. Driving started out as a wellness hindering activity and is now a wellness enhancing activity.

Another personal example of combining wellness areas I can

share is that I would love to ride bicycles with my wife. Unfortunately for me, she does not have the desire to ride a bike, ever. We tried and it didn't work. So we had to come up with a way we could spend leisure, fitness, and quality time together. We have chosen walking, and we make it a family event by going with our daughter and the dog. Coordinating this, I will admit, is challenging, but the main point in the wellness wheel approach is that we are moving in the right direction and we don't have to get it totally organized the first try. We can create all sorts of combinations if we focused our thoughts on it.

I could have pressed the issue of coaxing Dori into learning to ride a bike, but this will not work. The truth is, I rode my bike because I disliked walking. I used to see walking as an ineffective form of transportation that took too much time. Now I see walking as something wonderful. While listening to and reading the work of Dr. Andrew Weil, he so gracefully explained how walking is the easiest, safest, and most natural form of exercise there is. We were built to walk. We are supposed to walk. Also, at around the same time as I made a shift toward increasing my walking, we adopted an energetic dog who needed to be walked daily or he would tear the house down bit by bit. Because of this new attitude toward walking, I am able to enjoy walking for myself and for spending time with my family.

These were just examples of how you can organize your time to fit complete wellness into you life. I am sure that most schedule challenges you come up with as a no win situation, actually have a win-win solution if you search long enough. Whatever you do, do not sacrifice any wellness area for another, on a long term basis. I especially mean do not cut back on sleep to "fit-in" other things. Getting enough sleep will allow for enough energy and clarity to fulfill complete wellness.

Less is More

We live in such a busy and competitive culture, and we often make a game out of it. Except in this game, you get and keep points by collecting more stuff and taking on more tasks with less sleep and less time for yourself. And whoever can do this better, wins. But what do you really win by doing this? How much stuff is enough stuff?

I know a guy who is a compulsive gambler. He spends 80% of his time telling everyone about his stocks and his ups and downs in the market and with his bookmaker. I asked him the other day, "Hey J.K., when is enough money, enough money?" He looked at me with a very brief pause and said matter of fact, "It's never enough." I quickly responded, " Then that means you can never win." "That's right", he concurred. "Why play a game in which you can't win," I challenged. To this he had no answer.

In my parents house, they have four people living there, but for some reason they have six televisions. One in each bedroom, one in the living room, and one in the kitchen. The only other rooms left to put a television would be the bathrooms. Periodically they get new televisions, not because the old one was broken, but because they wanted a bigger one. Most people do not like to think they watch much television, because they are so busy doing other things. Well somebody is watching television because the statistics show this, and new television channels and shows are being created daily.

I have made a recent wellness change to cut back on 90% of my news intake. If there was something life altering I needed to absolutely be aware of, I would find out somehow, soon enough. Instead of eating breakfast with the morning news on TV, I turn on the radio and listen to a sports/entertainment show as a leisure activity, as the hosts usually make me smile, and I do like to follow sports somewhat. I honestly do feel more at ease, and I find I have more time for other things like reading, since going on this news fast.

More money does not necessarily mean more wellness. There will always be bigger and better material items you can possess. I am not going to tell you what to do with your money, however, I will suggest to explore the possibility of simplifying your life, in order to make more time for wellness. If you truly desired a stronger wellness circle, letting go of "stuff" and busy work should be a consideration. If you did not keep buying a new car every four years, maybe you could cut back on some overtime at work, in order to spend more time on exercise, which you keep telling everyone you don't have time for.

Getting out of debt should be a serious priority, in order to bring more wellness time into your world. Things like expensive jewelry and fancy clothes can be a part of a wellness lifestyle, only if you can afford to pay for them in cash. But if you keep buying and collecting "stuff" on credit, you will be blocking freedom. You might consider the benefits of canceling your cable TV service.(Oh no, I hope I didn't cross the line with this one.) I stopped watching music videos years ago, on purpose. I would rather create my own video with my imagination of what the song means to me, as opposed to what the song means to the producer. Cable TV can be addictive, it costs you money, and I even suppose it can lead to a repetitive strain injury of your thumb, secondary to constantly going through the one hundred and fifty channels, over and over.

The average income person has every bit of an opportunity for wellness as Bill Gates does. It all depends on where you choose to allocate your time. I am not discouraging anyone from dreams of being a millionaire, as I play the lottery every week, but being wealthy is not more important than my health, happiness, and longevity.

Making time for your family is something you can control. I love children, and sometimes I only want my daughter, and other times I feel like I want ten kids. (Depending on the time of day.) However, I fully realize the amount of time, energy, and money that is required to provide for my family. Therefore, making a decision to allow equal time for your wellness must be a consideration when starting a family. If I was independently wealthy, having ten kids would be an easier choice. But this is not the case at the time of this writing, and is not the case for many with this same decision.

Art Bell has a saying and a book called *The Quickening*. This is a term that represents the increasing speed at which our society and the environment operates from. Everything is built to go faster and faster so we can do more and more in the same twenty-four hours that we had one-hundred years ago. It is easy to get caught up with fast cars, fast communication methods and fast foods, so much so that we do not allow time for wellness. There are two definitions of the word *fast* in the dictionary. Maybe we should consider taking a fast from the fast lane of life, periodically, or definitely. You can control how fast or how slow you want to live your life. You do not have to get caught up in the *quickening* if you do not want to!

A few final notes on time. Stephen Covey has a fine approach to time management in his book *First Things First*, which will help you to see the big picture of principled time management. You may also consider studying the fields of quantum physics and metaphysics, to discover that time really doesn't exist after all. This would solve all of your time management challenges in an instant.

I feel safe in saying that you would have more time and opportunity for wellness if you let go of some of the "stuff" that may be clogging up your wellness wheel.

CHAPTER 12 LONGEVITY

It was Mickey Mantle who said, "If I knew I would have lived this long, I would have taken better care of myself." The problem is we do not know how long we will live. And when you are twenty years old, you have a feeling of immortality. You can do almost anything to your body/mind and it will forgive you immediately. But your bodymind stores up this abuse, until one day, the scales become too unbalanced and you fall hard.

Most people I have come into contact with like the idea of longevity, assuming they would be assured good health. I am sure you may have guessed by now what I am going to suggest. The answer is Yes! Developing your wellness wheel is the best way to ensure an optimal state of longevity.

Some people think they have the secret, like to consume mega-doses of vitamin C, daily exercise, or to eat the family's special longevity recipe. The answer is that all of these recipes may be correct because we are all unique, and may require certain key factors to create longevity, which may be different than your neighbor's key factors.

Scientists all over the world are working on various ways to alter the aging process, through cellular manipulation. They are working on ways of extending our life expectancy, but not necessarily our life span, which some say is fixed. This is certainly fascinating to explore, but at the time of this writing, no quick fix option seems within reach. Thoughts of longevity have been around for thousands of years, going back to Greek mythology and even to the bible in the book of Genesis, where reference is made to people living to be over nine-hundred years old. So maybe there is a lost key we are missing.

Genetics does play a role in longevity, but not much. If both parents or grandparents lived to be over eighty, you may only have an increased life expectancy of three years. And the most important thing to remember is that you cannot change your genetics. Maybe placing your concentration on what you can change, is the real missing link that scientists have been searching for.

What are some proven steps you can easily do to specifically increase your *chances* of a longer life. Remember, life is a game of odds, all you can ever do is to keep these odds in your favor. The following tips are very easy and sound suggestions for keeping longevity in your favor:

Own and care for a pet. Join a community service organization. Be a part of a support group. Eat less calories. You must be involved in a close relationship= marriage or roommate. Isolation = decreased longevity. Be surrounded by nature often. You must have strong spiritual beliefs. Eat breakfast every day. Maintain a steady and normal weight. Get eight hours of sleep. Don't smoke. Drink alcohol only in moderation if at all. Eat primarily a plant based diet. Being well educated proves for a longer life. If you are a woman, marrying a younger man favors longevity.

Where you live may definitely have an influence on longevity. The Vilcabamba of the Educadorian Andes, the Hunza of Pakistan, and the Abkazia in Soviet Georgia are all famous for generating centenarians. You do not have to go that far to get closer to longevity. People in Hawaii live longer than people in every other state in the United States, and the state of Utah has been rated to have the healthiest people in the U.S.. What do they all have in common? To me, all of these locations indicate that a simpler lifestyle with less "stuff" and with more exposure to nature from living in rural areas, is a factor in longevity. Moving to the suburbs is a good start in the right direction, but may not do as much for longevity as going "beyond the burbs."

I grew up in Daly City, which is the city that borders San Francisco to the southwest. San Francisco is a fun place to visit, but I would *never* live there. When I lived on the Big Island of Hawaii, I was absolutely able to see myself living to be a very happy old man. I saw clear stars in the sky at night. The ocean water was healthy and blue. The colors of the land were bright and plentiful. Rush hour traffic was non-existent, and no one honked horns at me or showed me their bird. I left my doors unlocked and "talked story" with my neighbors. Aloha flowed freely. My body/mind/soul was at peace. Certain family dynamics brought me back to California, which is where I will probably stay for a long time. I am in the suburbs now, and I do have plans within the next ten years to find a place, here in California, where I might find similar body/mind/soul peace.

Working with Longevity

I love to work with, and love to be surrounded by, my elders. I also love kids and get along great with them. My calling at this time is towards the people that I feel can teach me the most, which brings me happiness. In my work with the elderly, I evaluate them and ask routine questions. The following is what I consider to be a typical interaction.

I walk into the room slowly with a big smile, as I wave hello, stating my name and my job title. As she lies on her back with oxygen tubes in her nose, a bladder bag, and as she just finished swallowing ten different medications, I shout **"Why are you here?"** assuming she is hard of hearing.(Which she would let me know in a hurry if she was not.) This is a commonly asked question to determine a patient's orientation, not to be sarcastic. They usually respond, "I got sick." When I ask patients how they got sick, none of them have ever stated, "Because I live an unhealthy lifestyle." The patient usually pleads ignorance or they play the victim role, when asked how they got sick. As if everything was great and all of a sudden they got diabetes, atherosclerosis, hypertension, high anxiety, high cholesterol, and emphysema the day before they went to the hospital. Rarely do I find a patient who takes any responsibility for the predicament they are now in.

Part of an Occupational Therapy evaluation is to find out the patient's background and lifestyle, to help plan for their return to the highest functional performance level possible. Typical questions are the same ones I have in this book. "When do you exercise?" I often get a chuckle, which means they don't exercise at all. "What do you do for fun, for recreation?" I often hear, "Watch television I guess."(Which is the problem with the kids in America, they never fail to mention.) "What religious or spiritual practices do you have." "Not much anymore, I used to go to church, before my spouse died." I could go on and on, but I think you get the picture.

It may sound cruel, but I often ask myself, "What keeps these sort of people going, why don't they just call it quits and forget about the bilateral leg amputations at the age of eighty-nine? Why do they want chemotherapy at ninety-one for serious cancer? Is it because of the way they were brought up by their parents? Is it because they have not yet come to terms with death, and they are scared $h!tl~$$? Is it the human will and drive to fight until the end? This may seem like an arrogant question to ask, because I am a kid compared to a ninety-one-year-old, but I have, or at least *I think* I have, come to terms with my own eminent death and how I will handle it when it comes about. But how will I know when that time truly comes?

Why shouldn't the ninety-one-year-old cancer patient fight her disease if she feels it is not her time to go, and she needs to live to see another day. But for what, what does she want to see tomorrow that she cannot see today? If she were to miraculously beat this cancer and live to one-hundred-two years old, then got cancer again, and assuming she still had her wits about her, should she then go through the whole thing again? When does it end? What did she do differently during those eleven years? Probably not too much, as she was set in her ways.(As we will all be by then.) Yes she got to spend more time with her family, and perhaps more importantly, got to watch more of the "Price is

Right," dreaming about a date with the longevity blessed, Bob Barker.

Perhaps her inner intelligence is telling her to keep going, or maybe that same inner intelligence is telling her it is time to move on to a new level of being. This would be an interesting study indeed, to find out what the knower inside is really trying to tell those who are dying. Now this does not mean that as a therapist, I will not help these ninety- year-old's reach their goals, the best way I can. I have helped to send ninety-year-old's home, to live by themselves at a very independent functional level. And it is very gratifying work.

My great-grandmother, Zoe, is one-hundred-four years old at the time of this writing. She has lived in a nursing home for the past ten years, slowing declining in function that she can now barely move, hear, see, sleep, or eat, with no short term memory. And yet she still hangs on to life. But why? My sister thinks it is because Zoe is afraid of dying, and I think she is right. When she had her wits about her, Zoey would dance around the subject of God and death, so we never knew what she really believed.

I vividly remember when Zoe first went into the nursing home at age ninety-four. I left the building with tears falling from my eyes, saying to myself, "My grandmother does not belong here." From that day on, the main question I would ask myself is "What can I do to prevent anyone else's grandma from having to play out their years in living conditions like this."

Painful Aging

I hear young people, all the time, say that if they ever get in a state similar to that of my great-grandma's, that they would not do it. "Pull the plug--I don't want to live that long when my functions go--that's when it's time to call it quits," they say without hesitation. Fast forward fifty years, when these friends have long since lost many functions, and they now have a different perspective on life. They may now say, "It's not so bad, at least I can still talk and chew food."

I have yet to meet a person in a nursing home that intended on living there when they were younger. Do not think you are immune from ending up in one of these buildings some day. You may be no different than the people who live there now. The difference is that you can either take the messages I am proposing in this book to heart right now, or do you want to be confined to a wheel-chair at age seventy-four, kicking yourself in the butt repeatedly saying, " I should have read that Wellness For~Every~One book that all my healthy friends encouraged me to read when I was forty-one."

Each day we face decisions that may affect painful aging. Yesterday I went to the Giants baseball game, which I am trying to make a Father's Day tradition. It was the top of the ninth inning, and the Giants were losing 6-5 to the Cubs. The game was very long, it was starting to get very cold and windy, and we were all very tired. The attendance was over fifty-three thousand. We decided it would be better to leave the park now, in order to avoid having to wait in a traffic jam for an hour, and also knowing I had one-hundred miles to drive home that evening. We were able to get out of the parking lot with little trouble. We listened to the game on the radio on the ride home. The Giants made a terrific comeback in the bottom of the ninth to sweep the series.

There are two ways you could look at this situation. One is that I missed out on the excitement of the game's ending. The other way to look at it is that I prevented the future pain my family was in store for from having to deal with the large crowds of people leaving the building, fans driving crazy trying to beat everyone else out of the parking lot, getting stuck in stop-and-go traffic, the distress, etc. Sure it would have been nice to be there, with the majority of the crowd in the bottom of the ninth inning, but to me this is meaningless in the grand wellness scheme--the big picture.

You might be thinking "How does getting stuck in traffic have a relationship to aging." I will admit that on the surface it sounds silly, but remember your body has a tendency to store up all of the little abuses you subject it to over the years. Every time you got drunk, every time you "pigged out" at a holiday party, every time you got a severe sunburn, and every time you deprived yourself of sleep are all little pieces of the whole-synergistic-you. Some people follow the crowd at a young age in fear of missing out on life, but they forget that they may be decreasing their chances of being able to follow the crowd on a cruise to Alaska when they are eighty-two years old. Some people follow the crowd without regard for their own health.

When teenagers use drugs they are definitely operating from the here and now, following the crowd, focusing on how these drugs make them feel good in the moment, but they don't see the big picture. Thrill-seekers are the same way. They want the temporary rush of adrenaline, but they cannot hold this feeling for long, so they have to continue to seek thrills even at the expense of their lives. The big picture is that you can be in the here and now and feel good, and still see the big picture of wellness. This is what I am trying to teach. You do not have to race motorcycles or abuse drugs to feel good about yourself from an adrenaline high. You can be high on life by experiencing each moment as the miracle it is.

If you choose not to live anywhere near a wellness lifestyle, just realize how hard it will be for, and what a burden you will put on your family and friends. Your plans may be to live fast and die fast, that is, if you are lucky. However, I know first hand what the other side of the coin looks like, as I work with those who live fast and die slow. The pain it causes everyone to see their loved one lying there in the hospital, with tubes all over them, is a horrible experience. I have, as most medical staff personnel have, tried to become immune to these scenes, but it is not easy.

If the person is lucky, he will now see the light, change his ways, and fully recover from the stroke, heart attack, or shattered hip, and will not have to be a bother to anyone anymore. On the other hand, he may not be so lucky, with only little recovery. If this is the case, then his family and the government will have to take care of him for the rest of his life, at great stress and expense.

Is this what you want? Of course not, nobody wishes for this to happen. In fact I suppose many people at this moment are upset that I even mentioned this topic at all. I need to say it, and everyone else in the health field needs to start saying it.

YOU NEED TO START SAYING IT!

TAKE FULL RESPONSIBILITY FOR YOUR OWN WELLNESS!

Please understand that I am not saying you should blame yourself or that you should feel guilty about poor states of health. Blame and guilt are not a part of wellness. The next time you are faced with a health concern, you might consider saying the following:

"I have not been leading a balanced wellness lifestyle, which contributed to the compromised condition I am now experiencing. I will learn from this experience and concentrate my efforts on building my wellness circle, to prevent future discomforts."

I am not insensitive, I totally understand there are certain situations we have no control over, like someone born with a genetic disability, or a victim of a tragic accident. I am pleading to the ones who have the wonderful freedom of choice. The ones who know exactly what to do to minimize future painful experiences.

I would like to urge everyone, even if death is the hardest thing to think about, to at least write a will, establish a medical power of attorney, or have a living trust drawn up, today! The short term pain it may cause you now will absolutely save your family from possible years worth or grief. This way, your family does not have to decide what to do with your fate or your affairs. A thoughtful book I read on this subject is called *Peaceful Dying*, by Daniel Tobin M.D. It is simple to read, with good tips and insight.

Crampa

My grandfather(I say *crampa*, as I never stopped mispronouncing this word since childhood) had a massive stroke two weeks before my birth. He is still kicking, but since the stroke, he never went back to his career, he has expressive aphasia, and only has use of the left side of his body. Now don't get me wrong, he is a wonderful man and I sincerely love him, but I often wonder what it would have been like to know him without the effects of the brain attack. But then again, he was one of the reasons for inspiring me to become an Occupational Therapist.

Before the brain attack, my family tells me, he smoked cigarettes regularly, ate a high fat diet, and led a very stressful life. After the stroke, the whole family, my dad, me, and my brothers had to help him out with things he used to do for himself. Such as fixing his brakes.(Which we did many times a year, because he could still drive, and it was his favorite pastime. He drove with two feet, his right foot always stayed on the accelerator since he had little control over it, and his left foot would control the brake. So the brake pads always wore thin quickly as the brake was always trying to offset the accelerator.) We had to fix things around his house and do various other tasks. Again, don't misunderstand me, I would not trade any time I spent with him for anything. He is almost always smiling and I only have good memories about him. However, everyone would have loved to do the same things with him, but without the effects of the stroke.

We know history has a way of repeating itself, so I have been trying to point this fact out to my own father, usually in a subtle manner. I do not wish to spend my adult life caring for him after he has something that debilitates him because of factors he had total control of. I would rather go on vacations and to my child's ball games with him, instead of transferring him to the toilet three times a day. This is not my idea of fun. Again, do not get me wrong, if this unfortunate scenario did occur, I would help him without question, but I'd rather play golf.

He rationalizes that he never smoked and does not live a stressful life, therefore, he will not suffer the same fate as his father. However, he has had unstable cholesterol levels for many years, often in the three-hundred range. He does not exercise regularly, and his diet is not favorable, including large amounts of coffee in the day and wine at night. He has been very slow to make significant efforts to deal with this situation, with little progress, and I am afraid it will be too little--too late.

I wish I could say, so take care of yourself, get your wellness wheel rolling, and at least save your family from future unhappiness. But I cannot whole heartily say this, because I do not think it would work. I believe you need to be selfish when it comes to wellness. You have got to want it for yourself and not for others. This is the only way it will prove true. This is the only way to true happiness.

Prevention

The medical industry is a weird paradox. Professionals are trained to help people deal with their immediate problems first, and if there is time left over, which is rare, they can help people prevent these negative life events from happening again. Basically this is how we were taught in the West, whether you are a doctor, nurse, or therapist. We were taught how to repair the patient's problems, with little or no emphasis on prevention.

The medical business is like any other business. If the number of sick people in town goes down noticeably, then the need for skilled professionals is decreased. I have heard things from my peers like, "Things are so slow lately, I only have one or two patients to treat today." They say these things in a depressed manner. A lack of patients means they have to go home early with a smaller paycheck. I actually once heard someone say "Maybe a bus-load of people will fall off the road, then things will pick up."

Believe it or not, I actually see having a lack of patients to treat as a good thing. This is a strong indication that folks are healthy and do not need care. My peers always look at me cross-eyed when I tell them it would not bother me a bit if everyone across the land never needed any medical services again. "But then you would be unemployed," I would hear from a dissenter. I would only be unemployed temporarily, and then I would find a new way to contribute to the world. Somehow I feel I am in the minority with this point of view.

Another weird paradox is when a person, let's call him John, goes to a full rehabilitation hospital, let's say after having a stroke, he will have many different medical team members available to help him recover. The irony is that these members teach the patient about the same wellness areas I have discussed in this book.

First, you have the occupational therapist who trains John in the skills for the job/*career* of living, that he retired from two years ago. Then there is the physical therapist, who is trained to help John increase his *fitness* level, through walking, which Joe kept neglecting to do the past twenty years. Next, John gets to spend time with the recreation therapist, who allows him to participate in *leisure* activities while in the hospital. The same activities he probably wasn't doing at home. At night, John can push the call button to ask the nurse's assistant to bring him a pillow and a warm blanket to help him *sleep*, or to bring him *water* to swallow his sleeping pill. When John wants to discuss religion, the house chaplain will come by and broach the subject of *spirituality,* the subject John forgot about since the 1970's began. The hospital encourages plenty of *family and friends* to come and visit, even the ones that forgot to visit him the past five years. John's speech therapist will rehabilitate his *thought* processes and *communication* skills, as many stroke patients have difficulties expressing themselves, which John was never very good at to begin with. Do not forget the dietician, who will visit John to find out ways to provide proper *nutrition* while catering to his taste buds. And last but not least, there is the physiatrist, psychologist and registered nurse who are in charge of John's *body/mind,* by providing the correct medications and tests.

Wouldn't it make so much more sense to see all of these professionals **before** he had the stroke? Better still, how about listening to your intuition right now, and start to educate yourself to build a strong-balanced wellness circle. Building your wellness wheel is the same thing as building your ability to prevent harm. Doesn't it make more sense to spend a little time and a few bucks now to increase your wellness, as opposed to spending thousands of hours and dollars struggling with situations that are highly preventable?

I have recently started my own business. I decided I would rather spend a few hours with the people of the community, providing wellness education, instead of spending numerous hours providing rehabilitation services to them in the hospital. I have made this business as easy as possible. I provide a free wellness evaluation at the location of the client's choice, whether that means their home, place of business, or the local park. There is absolutely no obligation, no pressure, and I do not want to sell them any products. I felt if I took away the average person's usual excuses of not having enough time or money to seek out professional health education, then I could reach more people. This business is a new concept as far as I know.

The general population believes that simply getting an annual physical examination from their allopathic doctor is all they need to do to be assured of "good health." I am not suggesting that you refrain from continuing this practice. However, does your doctor examine all of your eight wellness areas, or does he/she merely examine your physical body? Does he find out what your spiritual beliefs are and where you get your wellness education from? Does she ask if you are making enough time for your favorite leisure activity or what you ate for dinner last night? The point is, do not fool your inner intelligence into assuming that everything is fine just because your blood test was within "normal" ranges. I foresee the day when insurance companies will not only pay for annual physicals, but they will also pay for annual wellness evaluations. But for now, you are the one that needs to go to the next step, beyond the annual physical exam.

I have spent enough time working with unhealthy people that I believe I know what the factors are that cause them to go to the hospital. Following the Wellness For~Every~One approach is now what I am contributing to my local community and to you the reader, to prevent harm and to live the life you want and deserve.

Our society is slowly catching on to the concept of wellness. We are going through a collective consciousness stage in regard to health right now. Soon we will reach the critical number of similar wellness thinking body-minds to tip the scales which will create a world-wind of health, happiness, and longevity. So for now, consider yourself to be a trend-setter as you grow further along the wellness road less traveled.

Living Forever

I think we all have a "goal-age" we see ourselves living to. I have this picture of myself at ninety-five years old, skiing down the slopes of "Heavenly Mountain," in South Lake Tahoe, from the highest peak(at least if I keel-over there, I will have a shorter commute) having all the youngsters stop and whisper, "Did you see that old guy going past me on the moguls?"

I would suggest to read up on the subject of longevity, which is easily available. Try Deepak Chopra's, *Ageless Body, Timeless Mind.* He presents bodymind blowing revelations that are fun to contemplate. One idea he proposes is to focus your awareness on the here and now, and not to worry about the fact that you are seventy-five years old, and how the clock is ticking faster. Animals do not spend their time worrying about getting gray hair, do they? Remember, you are what you think about all day long, so forget about your current age and think about how it feels to be twenty-one again, all day long. Also, consider giving your watch away, and instead, focus on your happiness today.

Taking care of *our* earth is definitely a part of a wellness lifestyle. If you fear being labeled an environmental wacko, just because you care about our ecology, do not worry. You can take care of the earth for selfish reasons. Deepak Chopra tells of an old story which reveals three gifts from the universe that: heal everyone equally, are free, and abundant. Those three things are: **sunlight, clean water, and a brisk walk in the fresh air.**

Although the subtitle of this book states *optimal health, happiness, and longevity for the 21st century*, maybe I should say for the 21st century and beyond. But if we want to experience a century full of wellness, we need to clean up our environment and concentrate on world peace. I know I keep suggesting the idea of focusing on the here and now, yet if we want to experience more here and nows in the future, it would make sense to concentrate on here and now topics that will also create more here and nows for centuries to come.(Was that a confusing sentence or what!)

I also know I harped on the benefits of breast milk, yet there

131

are recent reports of very toxic substances being found in breast milk as a result of poisons in the environment that humans absorb in their bodies. What good would it do to breast feed your child if you were feeding him/her toxins that would prevent wellness? If you truly want wellness for~every~one, caring for the earth is the same as caring for yourself and your family!!!

Striving for longevity is a part of wellness, only if your goal is to experience happiness to its fullest. Striving for longevity as a means to put off your eminent death, because of fear, is not related to wellness. If you come to positive terms with the death of your body and your physical life on earth, at an early age, your fears will dissipate and happiness will be the only option left. Being at peace with death does not mean that you obsess over it daily, this is not healthy. And remember, death is a natural occurrence, it is guaranteed and it is safe. Also, some cultures actually celebrate death.

I was once of the belief that we did not know life before we were born, and thus we will not know life after we are dead. Operating from this premise, my goal was to live as long as I could, because if I only lived once, I better experience everything possible before the last dance. This belief led to my thoughts of outliving everyone, which is one probable reason for my wellness mentality. As I have eluded to before, I am now moving toward the knowing that I did experience life before this life, and I will know life after this one is over. Maybe not in the form and name of James Dennis, but in another kind of form, yet to be remembered. This makes my life so much more fun and peaceful, that it is hard to describe.

Whichever reality is truth, is fine with me. For if there is no life after death, how could it be bad when death would mean eternal sleep, and you know how I feel about sleep.

My belief is that the healthier you are, the closer you are to God. To me it seems likely I will take my wellness with me when I go. I do not think it is likely I will take "stuff" with me after my last breath.

The Fountain of Youth is real, in that a strong wellness circle will carryover into the afterlife, only if this is your belief. I am not searching for the Fountain of Youth, for I know I have already found it, and shared it with you. You just read finished reading it!

Follow Up

Congratulations, you are now finished. Actually, you are only finished with this book, because as the title of this book indicates, wellness is forever. You now have the principles available to you, to create any level of wellness you desire.

At this point, I would like you to go back to your original wellness rating diagram. Go over each area, one by one, and ask yourself if you feel the numbers you chose are still accurate. Go ahead and erase the dashes and fill in new ones, if a new number is more appropriate. After you complete this, you do not necessarily have to fill out this diagram ever again, if you feel you have a good handle on the concept. Or you might want to start a fun tradition of pulling out this wellness circle diagram once a year, how about every January 1, and see where you are now balancing on the wellness scale.

Let's finish by saying the following aloud. Saying this phrase, or saying anything aloud can be very powerful because you cannot say something aloud without first having to think it, and it is our thoughts that help to shape our wellness destiny. Say it loud and proud:

"I am perfect exactly how I am right now, and I will make positive ongoing changes in my lifestyle to create maximum health, happiness and longevity."

Wellfully yours,
James Dennis

135

Appendix

Yesterday my wife was driving us home while I was reading Wayne Dyer's new book *Wisdom of the Ages*. In it he explores a poem written by Johann Wolfgang von Goethe titled *Lose This Day Loitering*. Seize not only the day, but rather, seize this minute, this moment, is the underlying theme of this poem. Goethe's poem can inspire you to get started on your wellness journey right now. Just get started and do not worry about what to do next or how it will end, because remember, ***wellness is never-ending***

Both Wayne and Goethe were pushing my inner self to put down that book and to pick up a pad and pencil, which was usually not available in this car. But I opened the glove compartment, and there was a pad and a pencil waiting for me the seize the moment. They were telling me to conclude my book with a self-written poem. I have never written a poem before, and I am not even sure that it is qualified to be considered a poem, but I am not bothered by that. Here it goes.....

Believe in Wellness

Can I believe wellness is a choice
If I already believe
I was not chosen to have wellness

How can I believe I am inherently perfect
If I already believe
I am a perfectionist

Should I believe there is no time like the present
If I already believe
I should be worrying about tomorrow's presents

Can I believe the sky is the limit
When I already know my limits

How can I believe balance is the key to life
When I believe
I should be searching for the key to life

Should I believe wellness in the 21st century is only a
heartbeat away
When I believe
A century full of heart surgeries has beat me today

Can I believe heavenly sleep is mine here on earth
If I believe
Sleep is for the weak that heaven doth seek

How can I believe nature heals us equally for free
When I am too busy believing
In deals and high heels and what's in it for me

Should I believe my soul is one with God forever
If I am forever waiting to see God

To believe or not to believe
Is what I believe
To be the question

James A. Dennis Jr.

Recommended Reading

Burton Goldberg Group. *Alternative Medicine*. Puyallup, WA: Future Medicine Publishing, Inc.,1994.

Campbell, Don. *The Mozart Effect*. New York: Avon Books, 1997.

Chopra, Deepak. *Ageless Body Timeless Mind: The Quantum Alternative to Growing Old*. New York: Harmony, 1993.

Coren, Stanley. *Sleep Thieves*. New York: Free Press, 1996.
Csikszentmihalyi, Mihaly. *Flow*. New York: Harper and Row, 1990.

Cutler, Howard. *The Art of Happiness*. New York: Riverhead Books, 1998.

Dyer, Wayne. *Your Erroneous Zones*. New York: Harper Paperbacks, 1976.

----------------- *Wisdom of the Ages*. New York: Harper Collins, 1998.

Fulford, Robert. *Dr. Fulford's Touch of Life*. New York: Pocket Books, 1996.

Galland, Leo. *The Four Pillars of Healing*. New York: Random House, 1997.

Grappo, Joseph. *Start Your Own Business in Thirty Days*. New York: Berkely Books, 1998.

Gray, John. *Men Are From Mars, Women Are From Venus*. New York: Harper Collins, 1992.

Hay, Louise. *You Can Heal Yourself*. Carlsbad, CA: Hay House, 1994.

Hirshberg, Caryle & Barasch, Marc Ian. *Remarkable Recovery*. New York: Riverhead Books,1995.

McDougall, John. *The McDougall Program*: *12 days to Dynamic Health*. New York: Plume, 1990.

Ornish, Dean. *Dr. Dean Ornish's Program For Reversing Heart Disease*. New York: Random House, 1990.

Pert, Candace. *Molecules of Emotion*. New York: Scribner, 1997. Robbins, Anthony. *Unlimited Power*. New York: Fawcett Columbine, 1986.

Robbins, John. *Diet for a New America*. Walpole, NH: Stillpoint, 1987.

Schultz, Mona Lisa. *Awakening Intuition*. New York: Harmony Books, 1998.

Tobin, Daniel. *Peaceful Dying*. Reading, Massachusetts: Perseus Books, 1999.

Walsch, Neale. *Conversation with God*. Charlottesville, VA: Hampton Roads, 1995.

Weil, Andrew. *Eight Weeks to Optimal Health*. New York: Knopf, 1997.

-------------------*Health and Healing*. Boston: Houghton Mifflin, 1983.

-------------------*Natural Health, Natural Medicine*. Boston: Houghton Mifflin, 1990.

--------------------*Spontaneous Healing*. New York: Knopf, 1995.
--------------------*Sound Body, Sound Mind*: *Music for Healing*. New York: Upaya, 1997.

About the Author

By trade, James A. Dennis Jr. is an Occupational Therapist who has worked in hospitals, skilled nursing facilities, and he especially loves home health care. Jim did not necessarily want to become an Occupational Therapist forever. What he really wanted was a diverse medical education which would allow him to help people in many regards. He has taken all of his knowledge and experience, while listening closely to his intuition to create his own niche in the health field.

Jim has started his own business which is intended to bring optimal health, happiness, and longevity to the people of his community and to the world. Although he enjoys providing rehabilitation services to people recovering from various illnesses, his true bliss is showing people how to prevent these illnesses from occurring in the first place. Initially he started to jot down a few notes to help organize his ideas into a working model. Though it was not his initial intention to write a book, he removed all inhibitions and started to write down his thoughts into a book format, which he is extremely proud of.

He has created a simple and balanced, yet powerfully effective approach with the Wellness For~Every~One theme. This is definitely one man who walks the wellness talk and is following the message his soul is longing to share, as he loves to speak to audiences about wellness. The future goal he is focusing on is his dream of becoming a renowned public speaker.

Mr. Dennis participates in various activities including golf, bike riding, and walking his dog. He loves spending quality time with his family, like when they go camping. Jim belongs to Toastmasters and a local service organization called Sertoma. He is a fun guy who always finds the humor in life, and he loves to meet new people as he greets them all with a big smile.

James A. Dennis Jr. is from the San Francisco Bay Area. He currently lives in Stockton California with his wife, daughter, dog, and parakeet.

You may contact him by E-mail: WellnessHC@hotmail.com

www.ingramcontent.com/pod-product-compliance
Lightning Source LLC
Chambersburg PA
CBHW020513290526
45786CB00002B/588